Dr. Golding on Hormone Basics

DR. CRAIGE GOLDING

These are the protocols and opinions of Dr Craige Golding.

Always consult your medical doctor before attempting to change or stop your medication.

Published by
The Golding Institute
65 Central Street
Houghton Estate
Johannesburg
2198

Written by Dr. Craige Golding
Editing by Lana Jacobsohn
Cover and layout by Dr. Carel-Piet van Eeden

Dr. Golding on Hormone Basics

CONTENTS

Foreword

OVER THE LAST TWENTY years the tide of anti-ageing medicine, with an emphasis on balancing the body's hormones and using the right nutrients, has started sweeping the globe. Because we live much longer the quest for living a healthier life has become a strong force.

It is an appropriate and almost natural phenomenon to see 'Bio-identical hormones made easy' appear from the pen of Dr Craige Golding.

At the turn of the century he became a futuristic pioneer for me and many medical practitioners in South Africa, who needed to expand their knowledge in the field of Integrative Medicine.

His teachings, wisdom and example reverberate through many medical practices all over our country benefiting thousands of people seeking to pursue health more than curbing illness.

As a specialist physician, his passion, integrity, and academic brilliance with his ever-expanding list of qualifications has earned him the right to be heard on any medical platform.

In addition to these audiences, the general public will benefit hugely from his practical and clear approach in this book.

He opens up the hormonal realm for any reader in his typical clear manner, instilling consciousness, whilst gently educating the reader through all the complexities. The exciting final part unfolds with practical solutions of how to live a long and healthy life by integrating bio-identical hormones and supplements into our daily lives.

The way I approach health, medicine, ageing and life as a medical doctor has been hugely changed by Craige Golding. I see the effect of this in patients on a daily basis and it makes me even more enthusiastic about the force this book will create in your dream for Healthy Ageing.

DR GYS DU PLESSIS

Introduction

BIO-IDENTICAL HORMONES MADE EASY!

In the years of practicing medicine, I have come across too many people struggling with their health and those who have been treated incorrectly for symptoms that are only a by-product of what is really going on with them.

Too many times it was as simple as bringing balance to their hormones.

Keeping your hormones in sync is one of the most important parts of making sure your body is functioning at its optimal level. Hormones like insulin and oestrogen are your body's chemical messengers. Slowly and quietly, they run through your bloodstream, regulating processes like growth, metabolism and mood.

Just one small change in hormone levels can cause a major imbalance, with side effects like fatigue, depression and weight gain.

While the number one way to keep your hormones in check is by consuming a variety of fresh, healthy foods on a daily basis, there are other things you can do that are very effective at keeping your endocrine system balanced.

That is why I'm writing this book so that I can bring clarity to those of you searching for an alternative to the conventional systems.

WHAT ARE HORMONES?

You have most likely heard of hormones at some point in your lifetime and may think you know what they do.

Well, the truth of the matter is that hormones and their function within the endocrine system are extremely complex.

There are multiple glands throughout the body, and each gland produces specific hormones designed to carry out certain functions. The whole process is actually quite amazing!

It also has the potential to be very overwhelming at times.

Whether you're premenopausal, postmenopausal or in-between – if you're tired of gulping ice water, gaining weight and suffering through endless mood swings…

Your life is about to change again - this time for the better!

The secret is creating a balance of two important body chemicals.

The first one is oestrogen - quite common. The second is one that gynaecologists don't even think to check!

If the balance of this vital hormone in your body is restored you may find that…

- You feel your body surge with energy
- Your muscle tone increases
- Your dry skin vanishes and looks fresher and younger… Even your wrinkles fade
- And you could enjoy the best orgasms ever!

It's true!

And there's so much more…

In this first-of-its-kind book on hormones you are about to learn a general overview of this highly important system and I will show you how to create the kind of lifelong health that will allow you to pursue your passions in life. You will look great, feel great, even lose weight, and have better sex.

To your good health

DR CRAIGE GOLDING
Specialist Physician
MBChB (Cum Laude) (Pret), FCP (SA)

MS USF, ABAARM, FAARFM

PART ONE

HORMONE AWARENESS

The worst thing you can do to a person with an invisible illness is to make them feel like they need to prove how sick they are.

CHAPTER 1

Some hormone history

T HERE'S A MYSTERIOUS SET of chemicals that flow through every part of your body. They can rule your life, govern your appetite, transform children into adults, and even affect your passion. They are called hormones and they are fundamental to making us who we are.

Hormones are absolutely fascinating because to a greater or lesser extent they control everything in your body.

The history of hormones it is a remarkable story that involves bizarre experiments with horrific wrong turns. Like the removal of young boys gonads to keep them from becoming men and so not letting their voices break or giving woman electroshock therapy to curb some of their menopausal symptoms.

But there have also been some extraordinary discoveries.

'The term 'hormone' was first used in 1896 by the Viennese gynaecologist Emil Knauer, who wrote of the existence of some 'mysterious chemical which controlled a variety of metabolic processes in the body.'

He named these chemicals 'hormones', from the Greek word hormao, to 'stir up' or 'incite'. A few years earlier, in 1889, Dr Edouard Brown-Séquard had announced that he was 'rejuvenated' after injecting himself with a mixture of guinea pig and dog testicle extracts. This led to a short–lived spell of interest into the research of sex-gland extracts as a possible source for a 'fountain of youth'.

In 1928, scientists at the University of Rochester in New York identified the ovarian hormone progesterone and its crucial role in preparing the uterus for pregnancy. The following year, the sex hormone oestrogen was isolated and identified by Dr Edward Doisy and Dr Edgar Allen at Washington University in St Louis. Together they established the existence of oestrogen and described its effects.

Once scientists had isolated progesterone and oestrogen, and determined their chemical structure, they explored their possible therapeutic effects, hoping that hormone treatments would be effective for gynaecological disorders.'[1]

Today, hormones are at the cutting-edge of medicine and their effects are more widespread than we have ever imagined.

Hormones are a crucial part of our biology and to better understand hormones is to better understand ourselves.

Our body has eleven systems that determine how we function:

ENDOCRINE SYSTEM

Endocrinology is the study of hormones. The endocrine system is what we call the 'working of hormones' in the body. It is the collection of glands that produce hormones that regulate:

- Metabolism
- Growth and development
- Tissue function
- Sexual function
- Reproduction
- Sleep
- Cognitive function and mood
- Body Temperature

The endocrine system is made up of a group of glands that produce the body's long-distance messengers, or hormones. Hormones are chemicals that control body functions, such as metabolism, growth, and sexual development. The glands, which include the pituitary gland, thyroid gland, parathyroid glands, adrenal glands, thymus gland, pineal body, pancreas, ovaries, and testes, release hormones directly into the bloodstream, which transports the hormones to organs and tissues throughout the body.

We have all heard about hormones but tend not to think about them every day. For something so fundamental to our lives, it's sad that it's the last of the systems to be fully understood.

Only at the turn of the 20th century did the medical world discover that the endocrine system is independent of the nervous system.

There are 80 known hormones in the human body and we'll take a closer look at the main ones in due course.

CIRCULATORY SYSTEM

The circulatory system is the body's transport system. It is made up of a group of organs that transport blood throughout the body. The heart pumps the blood and the arteries and veins transport it. Oxygen-rich blood leaves the left side of the heart and enters the biggest artery, called the aorta. The aorta branches into smaller arteries which then branch into even smaller vessels that travel all over the body. When blood enters the smallest blood vessels, which are called capillaries, found in body tissue, it gives nutrients and oxygen to the cells and takes in carbon dioxide, water, and waste. The blood, which no longer contains oxygen and nutrients, then goes back to the heart through veins. Veins carry waste products away from cells and bring blood back to the heart, which pumps it to the lungs to pick up oxygen and eliminate waste carbon dioxide.

DIGESTIVE SYSTEM

The digestive system is made up of organs that break down food into protein, vitamins, minerals, carbohydrates, and fats, which the body needs for energy, growth, and repair. After food is chewed and swallowed, it goes down the oesophagus and enters the stomach, where it is further broken down by powerful stomach acids. From the stomach the food travels into the small intestine. This is where the food is broken down into nutrients that can enter the bloodstream through tiny hair-like projections. The excess food that the body doesn't need or can't digest is turned into waste and is eliminated from the body.

IMMUNE SYSTEM

The immune system is our body's defence system against infections and diseases. Organs, tissues, cells, and cell products work together to respond to dangerous organisms (like viruses or bacteria) and substances that may enter the body from the environment. There are three types of response systems in the immune system: the anatomic response, the inflammatory response, and the immune response.

The anatomic response physically prevents threatening substances from entering the body. Examples of the anatomic system include the mucous membranes and the skin. If substances do get by, the inflammatory response goes on attack.

The inflammatory system works by excreting the invaders from your body. Sneezing, runny noses, and fever are examples of the inflammatory system at work. Sometimes, even though you do feel well, your body is fighting illness.

When the inflammatory response fails, the immune response goes to work. This is the central part of the immune system and is made up of white blood cells, which fight infection by gobbling up antigens. About a quarter of white blood cells (called the lymphocytes), migrate to the lymph nodes and produce antibodies, which fight disease.

LYMPHATIC SYSTEM

The lymphatic system is also a defence system for the body. It filters out organisms that cause disease, produces white blood cells, and generates disease-fighting antibodies. It also distributes fluids and nutrients in the body and drains excess fluids and protein so that tissues do not swell. The lymphatic system is made up of a network of vessels that help circulate body fluids. These vessels carry excess fluid away from the spaces between tissues and organs and return it to the bloodstream.

MUSCULAR SYSTEM

The muscular system is made up of tissues that work with the skeletal system to control movement of the body. Some muscles—like the ones in your arms and legs—are voluntary, meaning that you decide when to move them. Other muscles, like the ones in your stomach, heart, intestines and other organs, are involuntary. This means that they are controlled automatically by the nervous system and hormones—you often don't even realise they're at work.

The body is made up of three types of muscle tissue: skeletal, smooth and cardiac. Each of these has the ability to contract and expand, which allows the body to move and function. .

Skeletal muscles help the body move.

Smooth muscles, which are involuntary, are located inside organs, such as the stomach and intestines.

Cardiac muscle is found only in the heart. Its motion is involuntary.

NERVOUS SYSTEM

The nervous system is made up of the brain, the spinal cord, and nerves. One of the most important systems in the body, the nervous system is your body's control system. It sends, receives, and processes nerve impulses throughout the body. These nerve impulses tell your muscles and organs what to do and how to respond to the environment.

There are three parts of the nervous system that work together: the central nervous system, the peripheral nervous system, and the autonomic nervous system.

The central nervous system consists of the brain and spinal cord. It sends out nerve impulses and analyses information from the sense organs, which tell the brain about things you see, hear, smell, taste and feel.

The peripheral nervous system includes the cranio-spinal nerves that branch off from the brain and the spinal cord. It carries the nerve impulses from the central nervous system to the muscles and glands.

The autonomic nervous system regulates involuntary action, such as heartbeat and digestion.

REPRODUCTIVE SYSTEM

The reproductive system allows humans to produce children. Sperm from the male fertilises the female's egg, or ovum, in the fallopian tube. The fertilised egg travels from the fallopian tube to the uterus, where the foetus develops over a period of nine months.

RESPIRATORY SYSTEM

The respiratory system brings air into the body and removes carbon dioxide. It includes the nose, trachea, and lungs. When you breathe in, air enters your nose or mouth and goes down a long tube called the trachea. The trachea branches into two bronchial tubes, or primary bronchi, which go to the lungs. The primary bronchi branch off into even smaller bronchial tubes, or bronchioles. The bronchioles end in the alveoli, or air sacs. Oxygen follows this path and passes through the walls of the air sacs and blood vessels and enters the blood stream. At the same time, carbon dioxide passes into the lungs and is exhaled.

SKELETAL SYSTEM

The skeletal system is made up of bones, ligaments and tendons. It shapes the body and protects organs. The skeletal system works with the muscular system to help the body move.

Marrow, which is soft, fatty tissue that produces red blood cells, many white blood cells, and other immune system cells, is found inside bones.

URINARY SYSTEM

The urinary system eliminates waste from the body, in the form of urine. The kidneys remove waste from the blood. The waste combines with water to form urine. From the kidneys, urine travels down two thin tubes called urethras to the bladder. When the bladder is full, urine is discharged through the urethra.

HOW WELL-INFORMED ARE WE?

What we knew about hormones, even as little as 10 years ago, has changed dramatically.

With everyone having access to Google and the internet there is an information overload.

You all know what I mean, in the simplest form… Facebook is full of it.

'Don't drink coffee because it's not good for you.' Then next week or even the next day you're told to drink coffee because it's good for you as it helps stimulate your metabolism.

As was the case with smoking, it was an accepted part of society years ago, but now people who smoke are shunned in social environments. Never mind the chances of contracting lung cancer or heart disease.

The point I'm trying to make has nothing to do with coffee and cigarettes.

The point is, the medical field moves at such a fast pace with new discoveries, and new results based on years of studies, are being released almost daily.

This is especially true when it comes to hormones.

What happened in the past?

When my mother was young, if a woman had a hysterectomy, she was immediately put on hormone replacement therapy.

This was revolutionary at the time, but now it has been discovered that the artificial hormones women were taking were causing lasting bone density loss, thyroid problems and even Type 2 diabetes.

If we go back even further, doctors often removed women's ovaries in the hope of stopping depression, nymphomania, hysteria and what was referred to as "women's ailments".

Despite the advances how much do we really know?

Even with the advances in technology we have today with regard to e-mail, there are still people wanting to communicate by letter or telephone. A similar thing happens with many doctors.

There is so much to know and so much conflicting information out there that you need to educate yourself with the help of a trusted hormone expert.

CHAPTER 2

What are hormones?

CLEARING UP THE CONFUSION

Let's take a closer look at how the endocrine system works.

Hormones are our body's chemical messengers that send messages from one place to another. One thing people don't usually realise is that the brain is totally involved in this whole process.

It starts with a message from the hypothalamus, which is an area of the brain responsible for the production of many of the body's essential hormones. The hypothalamus makes what are called releasing hormones.

These hormones go to the pituitary gland, a section of the brain responsible for controlling growth and development and the functioning of the other endocrine glands. The pituitary gland makes what they call stimulating hormones.

The stimulating hormones are released from the pituitary gland to other glands in the body.

The glands might be the ovaries, testicles, adrenals or thyroid.

All of these different glands are activated by the stimulating hormones, and that causes the receiving gland to release its own hormones – which can either be testosterone, progesterone, oestrogen, thyroid hormones or adrenal steroids.

The really interesting part is that these hormones go into what we call a 'feedback loop' and they act upon the hypothalamus. So if there's more than enough of a particular hormone in the blood, the message that goes back to the hypothalamus is 'slow down the releasing hormone'. It slows down the whole system, stopping any release of hormones from the different glands.

So the hormone released from the brain acts like a messenger boomerang.

It's a whole cycle that happens continually in our bodies while we carry on unaware.

Another thing about hormones that is really important to understand is that not only is there this whole feedback loop, but there is also the balance of hormones and how hormones work together in the body.

Certain hormones affect other hormones, negatively and positively

When we have too much of a particular hormone in our blood it can stop other hormones from sending messages to the correct glands and can stop them from working completely.

The same can occur if you have too little.

There's a very complex interplay between different hormones. What we really need is all the hormone messages to be in balance and to work together.

A few hormones and their function:

- **Insulin** from the pancreas tells the cells to take up glucose from the blood to use as energy.
- **Thyroxin** from the thyroid gland speeds up the metabolism of cells generating energy and burning fat.
- **Oestrogen and progesterone** from the ovaries control a sequence of changes that maintain fertility and the menstrual cycle.

THE POLITICS OF HORMONES

There are three classifications of hormones: Amino acids, Lipids and Peptides.

Hormones are:

- Fat-like amino acids, called steroid hormones, that absorb into the cells
- Protein-like lipids such as insulin which are absorbed through the cell wall, and
- Peptide hormones are stored in fluid-filled pockets in the cell until the proper stimuli signal release into the bloodstream which will activate the absorption.

The absorption of the different types of hormones can happen at the same time like a domino effect, called hormone cascade. Pathways are usually regulated by negative feedback as hormone cascades.

It's like a symphony!

If you have the piano section missing and the base section missing, the music just wouldn't be as full and as rich.

When you have all of the sections functioning together, it makes beautiful music.

When all of the hormones are balanced, that's when you feel your absolute best.

CHAPTER 3

Hormone overload

WHO IS THE CONDUCTOR OF THE HORMONE SYMPHONY?

Each part of your body from your brain to your skin, your heart, your kidneys, and your muscles all have specific jobs.

They take direction from your endocrine system to get the work done.

The glands of the endocrine system send out hormones that tell each part of your body what work to do, when to do it, and for how long.

ENDOCRINE SYSTEM... SAY WHAT?

As mentioned, the endocrine system consists of several glands, all in different parts of the body, which secrete hormones directly into the blood.

Hormones have many different functions and modes of action. One hormone may have several effects on different target organs or the target organ may be affected by more than one hormone.

But how do our hormones and endocrine system get disrupted?

Endocrine System

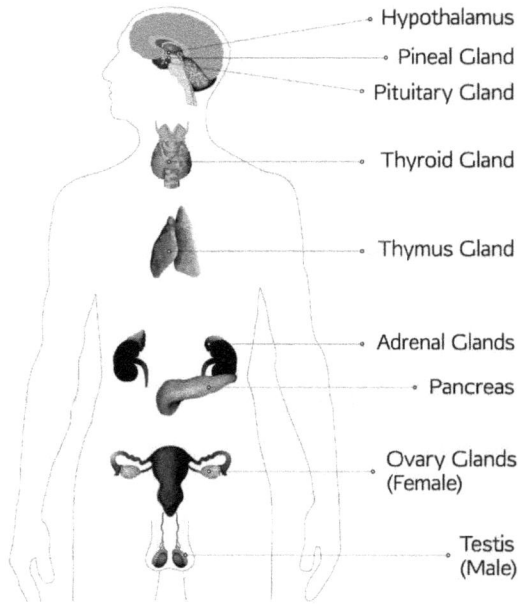

- Hypothalamus
- Pineal Gland
- Pituitary Gland
- Thyroid Gland
- Thymus Gland
- Adrenal Glands
- Pancreas
- Ovary Glands (Female)
- Testis (Male)

The endocrine system

CHEMICALS FUEL HORMONE OVERLOAD

These are chemicals known as hormone disruptors. Fifty years ago, these were not considered an issue because the food eaten by our grandparents was mostly organic. But in the world we live in today, with so much processed food and other harmful chemicals, our health is under real threat.

Some of the symptoms of hormone overload are:

- Weight gain
- Fatigue

- Anxiety
- Joint pain
- Chronic diseases, like cancer

We all have one or more of these symptoms at any given time. This is because endocrine disruptors maintain how we feel at least 80% of the time.

HELP! Toxins!

Lurking inside many foods are dangerous substances such as:

Toxins are a class of chemicals that imitate hormones. A surge in these hormone-like chemicals is impacting our health and environment in a profound way. Household cleaning products are getting washed into our natural water systems and are being absorbed into our soils and spilling into oceans where they affect marine life. Never mind the risk inside your home when you inhale and absorb these toxins.

Pesticides are being sprayed over vegetable and fruit crops daily. These are then absorbed into the soil and affect next season's crop harvest...a vicious, ongoing cycle.

BPA/Plastics and preservatives in beauty products like shampoo and body cream. There are many harmful chemicals in the plastic containers.

These toxins hide in stored fat in your body. What you need is a way to clean up the metaphoric streets in your blood from these disruptors.

HOW DO ENDOCRINE DISRUPTORS WORK?

Researchers have learned much about the mechanisms through which endocrine disruptors influence the endocrine system and alter hormonal functions.

Endocrine disruptors are chemicals that interfere with the body's endocrine system and produce adverse developmental and larger problems in the reproductive, neurological and immune systems. They are mostly to blame for hormone imbalance.

Endocrine disruptors can:

Mimic or partly mimic naturally occurring hormones in the body like oestrogens and progesterone (the female sex hormones), androgen (the male sex hormone), and thyroid hormones; producing overstimulation.

They can also bind to a receptor within a cell and block the endogenous hormones from binding. The normal signal then fails to occur and the body fails to respond properly. Examples of chemicals that block or antagonise hormones are anti-oestrogens and anti-androgens.

Lastly, they can interfere or block the way natural hormones or their receptors are made or controlled, for example, by altering their metabolism in the liver.

CHAPTER 4

The rise of hormone related problems

A BETTER UNDERSTANDING OF TOXIN disruptors has, in turn, come with an increase in understanding of the endocrine system and medical advancements in this field.

But what are we left with if we know how things work but we can't keep ourselves healthy?

You're almost guaranteed to know someone with a serious illness such as obesity, diabetes, heart disease or cancer. My waiting room is full of men and women who are battling with such diseases.

The disease may vary but the cause stays the same.

A new United Nations report has provided more evidence linking endocrine disrupting chemicals to the development of different cancers, obesity and diabetes.

The report State of the Science of Endocrine Disrupting Chemicals by the United Nations

Environment Programme (UNEP) and the World Health Organization (WHO) says that there is a growing probability that maternal, foetal and childhood exposure to chemical substances plays a larger role in causing endocrine-related diseases and disorders.

'We present new proofs that there is a link between endocrine disrupting chemicals and common diseases,' Åke Bergman, professor at Stockholm University and chief editor of the report, said in a statement.

Endocrine illnesses are so common and on the increase, we can see the link to endocrine disrupting chemicals. The rate of the increase is so great that genetic causes can't be the reason why.

In the report, the researchers show there are several disorders which are increasing and can be linked to endocrine disrupting substances:

Cancer – breast cancer, endometriosis, prostate cancer, testicular cancer and thyroid cancer increase.

Obesity and diabetes have increased over the past 40 years, especially Type 2 diabetes, which has more than doubled since 1980.

Decreasing male sperm counts and genital malformations are increasing among young boys.

Let's take a look at the potential problems

These are the problems that occur most often and the ones I help treat again and again.

CANCER

Endometrial cancer is having too much of the hormone oestrogen, compared to the hormone progesterone, in the body. This hormone imbalance causes the lining of the uterus to thicken. If the lining builds up and stays that way, then cancer cells start to grow.

Testosterone actually protects against prostate cancer, but if our bodies can't stop the effects of increased oestrogen, testosterone will decline and the development of prostate cancer will occur.

Breast cancer develops from higher levels of oestrone present in your body. These are produced by toxins causing imbalance which results in more breast-cell stimulation. Higher levels of oestriol present in your body means less breast-cell stimulation protecting you.

- Oestriol = Good. Oestrone = Bad.

DIABETES

Diabetes is a chronic disease that interferes with the body's ability to use glucose for energy. It is caused by problems with the hormone insulin, but it can also be affected by other hormones like the stress hormone cortisol, causing overproduction of adrenaline, thyroid hormone and growth hormone.

HEART DISEASE

Oestrogen causes water retention that increases blood pressure. High blood pressure increases the risk of both heart attacks and strokes. A normal blood pressure irrespective of age should be 120/80. A healthy cholesterol level should be 190 -210mg/dl. Oestrogen also accelerates the ageing of collagen, weakening the walls of the arteries.

DEMENTIA & DEPRESSION

Research has shown repeatedly that patients with dementia have low levels of T3 thyroid hormone. Endocrine disrupters are a main cause in dementia in young and old people. Elevated cortisol levels are leading to cognitive impairment and a cause of depression. Low levels of melatonin and serotonin hormones produced by your brain play a large role in dementia and especially depression.

INFERTILITY & LOW SEX DRIVE

Polluted environments have wreaked havoc with human fertility. Not only has the average sperm count dropped by more than 50% in the West, but endocrine disruptors have affected women's fertility from as early as her time *in utero*. Too little testosterone in men and women from too much oestrogen, causes a drop in sex drive.

HORMONES AND RELATED DISEASES

Pioneering research, over the past 50 years, has been done by the National Institute of Environmental Health Sciences on the health effect of endocrine disruptors.

They have proved over and over again that diseases are caused from the amount of chemicals, pesticides, herbicides and hormone oestrogen being pumped into our food, water supplies, and ironically, even in the pills we take to help us stay healthy.

The rise of serious illnesses is a 20th century pandemic that is widespread across the world. The western medical profession is dominated by doctors who prescribe non-identical hormone replacements that are full of synthetic oestrogens or anti-depressants which often just repress underlying issues whilst not dealing with the cause.

You have the choice, there are a range of treatments that can, and do work.

PART TWO

HORMONES: THE FACTS

If you listen to your body when it whispers,
you won't have to hear it when it screams.

CHAPTER 1

Tracking and interpretation

S IGNS AND SYMPTOMS OF hormone imbalance are so vast that many times they are not immediately picked up or diagnosed correctly.

Your most powerful ally in reaching your goal of hormone balance and optimal health is you. It's ultimately up to you to educate yourself and keep track of how you're doing.

It will help you to monitor your symptoms before taking any supplements or bio-identical hormones; or alter your dose if any symptoms return.

Maintaining hormone balance is more than just taking the right hormones at the right times in the correct dosages. Many aspects of your lifestyle, from diet and exercise, to stress and sleep patterns, can impact your hormone levels.

Common signs and symptoms of hormonal imbalance in men and women

IN WOMEN

SLEEP DISORDERS

You may find it hard to fall asleep just before your period. This may be due to the sharp drop in the hormone progesterone. Progesterone has relaxing properties, so when its levels drop, it can make you feel restless and cause your sleep disorders.

Progesterone levels also drop after giving birth, but then you can always blame your baby if you are not getting enough sleep.

Progesterone levels drop as you go through menopause.

PERSISTENT ACNE

You can have a breakout before your period, due to hormonal shifts. However, if you suffer from deep, cystic acne all the time, then it could be androgens (male hormones such as testosterone) which are the culprit. Testosterone stimulates excess production of sebum (oil), which then gets trapped underneath the skin and merges with acne-causing bacteria and dead skin cells. That leads to clogged pores, pimples and blemishes. The higher a woman's testosterone levels are, the worse the breakout.

MEMORY FOG

Are you forgetting things? Such as where you put your handbag, or what time you're meant to meet your friend? If so, then this could be a hormonal issue. If you've been experiencing a high amount of stress recently, then your body will be producing high levels of the stress hormone cortisol. Studies suggest that consistently high levels of cortisol can dull your learning ability and memory.

CONSTANT HUNGER

It's important to eat healthily and exercise. It may be because of your hormones that you are so ravenous. Are you getting enough sleep? In one study, volunteers who were deprived of sleep saw their levels of the hormone ghrelin soar — making them extremely hungry — while their levels of the hormone leptin plummeted. You see, ghrelin stimulates the appetite, whereas leptin and oxyntomodulin suppress it. This indicates why people who are chronically sleep-deprived (getting less than seven hours a night) tend to be more overweight than those who get more sleep.

DIGESTIVE PROBLEMS

The stress hormones affect us in different ways. Some people may carry stress in their heads and get tension headaches; some may just feel cranky and want to curl up on the sofa with a box of chocolates. However, some people carry stress in their stomach.

Cortisol production is naturally high in the early morning to help you wake up. However, people who chronically stress their adrenal glands to overproduce cortisol, alter their cortisol concentrations so that cortisol is low in the morning when they wake up, instead of high.

If you suffer from irritable bowel syndrome (IBS) it could be due to abnormal levels of serotonin. 90% of sufferers are women, some whose IBS symptoms flare up around menstruation. The flux of oestrogen and progesterone may also play a role.

CONSTANT FATIGUE

We all have days when we're so tired that we're desperate for a nap. However, if you feel exhausted every day, then you could be suffering from a lack of a thyroid hormone, a condition called hypothyroidism. It is more likely that you have this condition if you have gained 10 – 20kg which you cannot shift, even through diet and exercise. Thyroid hormones control the body's metabolism, and when the hormone levels are low, all systems slow down, including heart rate, mental functioning, and digestion. That's why hypothyroidism can make a person feel exhausted, mentally foggy, and even constipated.

MOOD SWINGS AND DEPRESSION

The onset of perimenopause and menopause result in a variety of physical and emotional symptoms causing stress, frustration, and ultimately depression.

You may experience mood swings, anxiety and lose your lust for life. It's common for menopause to prompt emotions of sadness and depression in women. It's estimated that between 8% and 15% of women in menopause experience depression in some form, often beginning in perimenopause.

The hormone imbalance associated with perimenopause and menopause inhibits your body from managing symptoms mentioned above.

WEIGHT GAIN

As women age, they tend to believe that putting on weight is inevitable. But there might be an underlying problem to such weight gain. The problem could be your adrenal system becoming fatigued and then signalling to your thyroid that there is a problem. Your thyroid then responds by slowing down your metabolism. The pancreas also responds to the signal by thinking it needs to conserve fat, and concentrates on storing fat in your mid-section, on your back and other places that are not suited to your particular body type.

HEADACHES AND MIGRAINES

As you enter middle age you may find that you suffer from frequent headaches and even migraines. This could be due to hormonal imbalances around certain times of the menstrual cycle. If you suffer from headaches and migraines, it could be helpful to keep a diary of when they occur. In this way, you can work out if they occur randomly, or if they seem to follow certain triggers.

HOT FLUSHES AND NIGHT SWEATS

It was once thought that being too low in oestrogen was the issue. However, we now understand that the cause may also be too much oestrogen and too little progesterone, or other hormone imbalance in your body that comes from the adrenals, ovaries, thyroid, pancreas, or gastrointestinal tract. These systems do not always stay in balance, and women are more prone to hormonal imbalances as they go through midlife changes.

VAGINAL DRYNESS

As menopause approaches, the reduction of oestrogen levels cause changes to the vaginal wall. This can cause vaginal dryness, which can make sex uncomfortable.

BREAST CHANGES

As women age high levels of oestrogen can make breasts feel tender and sore which could lead to lumps, fibroids, and cysts. That's why it is important to have annual examinations and screening mammograms. Get to know your breasts best by getting into the habit of checking yourself for lumps or anything unusual. While not every lump or breast change indicates cancer, it's still best to be on the safe side and talk to your doctor if you feel something suspicious.

LOSS OF LIBIDO

Hormonal imbalances can cause women to experience a low sex drive. This could be due to low levels of oestrogen and testosterone.

IN MEN

Many of the symptoms of male hormonal imbalances come on very gradually. You may not notice them at first, but as more symptoms appear and become worse over time, they do become obvious. The symptoms are some of the most common and are similar to those that women go through but with men it's mostly due to a loss of testosterone:

- Erectile dysfunction, fewer spontaneous erections and a low libido
- Difficulty achieving an orgasm and a reduced amount of semen with each ejaculation.
- Hair loss all over the body - not just on your head.
- Fatigue or lack of energy - loss of motivation and decreased passion for work, relationships or just life in general.
- Memory loss - difficulty remembering things and an inability to concentrate.
- Mood swings or increased irritability and nervousness - even depression or anxiety.
- Heart palpitations and cardiovascular risks.
- Muscle loss or weakness - a dramatic reduction in muscle size and strength.
- Sleep apnoea, insomnia, night sweats or hot flushes
- Increased body fat and the development of man breasts.

Men in andropause (male menopause) can also experience a lowered sperm count and a reduction in the proportion of red blood cells in their plasma.

People often mistake the symptoms of imbalanced hormones in men with signs of ageing.

Low testosterone is not often recognised and is undertreated. According to a recent estimate only 5% of men with low testosterone receive treatment.

HOW TO TRACK AND INTERPRET YOUR SYMPTOMS

Keeping track of your symptoms will give you and your doctor a very good general overview of what hormonal imbalance may be causing your symptoms.

Rate your symptoms (listed on the chart) on a scale of 0 – 5 DAILY FOR A MONTH.

0 – Not a problem

1 – Rarely a problem

2 – Bothers me occasionally

3 – Regularly a problem

4 – Almost always a problem

5 – Constantly a problem

Symptom	1	2	3	4	5	6	7	8	9	10	11	12	13	14	15
Aches & pains															
Acne, oily skin															
Allergies															
Anxiety															
Breast tenderness															
Breast lumps															
Cold hands and feet															
Decreased sex drive															
Depression															
Dry eyes															

Symptom	1	2	3	4	5	6	7	8	9	10	11	12	13	14	15
Dry skin															
Dry, brittle hair															
Endometriosis															
Fat gain															
Fatigue															
Foggy thinking															
Gallbladder pain															
Hair loss															
Headaches															
Heart palpitations															
Hot flushes															
Low blood sugar															
Insomnia															
Irritability															
Memory loss															
Migraines															
Muscle weakness															
Night sweats															
Osteoporosis															
Ovarian cysts															
Oversensitivity															
Painful intercourse															
Sleepiness															
Sluggish digestion															
Thinning skin															

Symptom	1	2	3	4	5	6	7	8	9	10	11	12	13	14	15
Talking excessively															
Bladder infection															
Vaginal dryness															
Weepiness															
Weight gain															

Other factors to track are:
- Meals, breakfast/lunch/dinner and snacks
- Water and other beverages like coffee/tea/alcohol
- Sleep: What time you go to bed and if it's constant. What time you wake up, and how many hours you have slept
- Vitamins & supplements
- Exercise
- Medication - over the counter and prescription
- Recreational activities
- Stressors
- Exposure to toxins
- TV viewing
- Relationships

SYMPTOMS AND THEIR POSSIBLE CAUSES

In the following list of symptoms you will be able to identify the possible cause of which hormones might be out of balance.

ACHES AND PAINS

- Low cortisol
- Oestrogen dominance
- Low testosterone

ACNE AND OILY SKIN

- High testosterone

ALLERGIES

- Oestrogen dominance
- Low cortisol
- Deficiency of Vitamin C and bioflavonoid

ANXIETY

- Oestrogen dominance
- Too much caffeine (coffee or soft drinks)
- Diet pills
- Deficiency of B Vitamins
- Chronic stress
- Too much TV

BREAST TENDERNESS

- Oestrogen dominance
- Too much caffeine

Supplementing with oestrogen, testosterone, DHEA or pregnenolone can create excess oestrogen and cause breast tenderness.

COLD HANDS AND FEET

- Oestrogen dominance interfering with thyroid function
- Low thyroid hormone levels
- Poor circulation caused by excess sugar in the diet
- Insulin resistance

DECREASED SEX DRIVE

- Low testosterone
- Oestrogen dominance
- Stress

DEPRESSION

- Both high and low oestrogen can contribute to depression
- Low progesterone

DRY EYES

- Oestrogen dominance
- Low testosterone

DRY SKIN

- Oestrogen deficiency
- Oestrogen dominance creating low thyroid function

ENDOMETRIOSIS

Caused by exposure to xenoestrogens (oestrogens that are foreign to the body, found in pesticides and plastics) in the womb and made worse by oestrogen dominance.

ABDOMINAL FAT

In menopausal women, oestrogen is both made and maintained by belly fat. However, too much abdominal fat is not good for the heart.

At what point or size does "good" belly fat become "bad" belly fat? It's quite natural for postmenopausal women to have a little bit of a belly, but more that that is usually an indicator of insulin resistance and/or high cortisol. The best way to tell whether it's helpful or harmful is simply by how it looks; an insulin-resistant belly is noticeably out of proportion to the rest of the body even in someone who is obese.

FAT GAIN

Excess fat around the hips, buttocks, and thighs is a hallmark symptom of oestrogen dominance.

Excess fat around the middle is usually a sign of insulin resistance (too much sugar and refined carbohydrates and too little exercise).

A poochy tummy (which is different from weight gain around the middle and different from the saggy tummy caused by pregnancy) can be caused by excess cortisol (stress), and/or oestrogen deficiency, and/or constipation.

FATIGUE

- Low cortisol
- Oestrogen dominance
- Stress
- Lack of sleep
- Chronic infection

- Poor diet (which can cause hypoglycaemia, a condition where blood sugar drops dramatically between meals).

FIBROCYSTIC (LUMPY) BREASTS
- Oestrogen dominance

Supplements with oestrogen, testosterone, DHEA or pregnenolone can create excess oestrogen and cause lumpy breasts.

FOGGY THINKING
- Low oestrogen
- Low testosterone
- Oestrogen dominance
- Hypoglycaemia (low blood sugar)

GALLBLADDER PAIN
- Excess oestrogen
- Oestrogen dominance
- Too much fat in your diet (especially fried foods)

HAIR LOSS
- Excess testosterone / male hormones (usually caused by excess sugar and refined carbohydrates in your diet)
- Excess oestrogen
- Oestrogen dominance
- Thyroid deficiency

HEADACHES
- Oestrogen dominance

HEART PALPITATIONS
- Low cortisol
- Low testosterone
- Low blood pressure
- Food allergy
- Stress

HOT FLUSHES
- Low oestrogen
- Low progesterone
- Fluctuating hormones caused by menopausal and andropausal transition

HYPOGLYCAEMIA (LOW BLOOD SUGAR)
- Oestrogen dominance
- Low cortisol

INCONTINENCE
(wetting pants when laughing, coughing or sneezing)
- Overall low hormones, especially common among women who have had a hysterectomy
- Obesity

INSOMNIA

It is not at all unusual for women and men going through the menopausal and andropausal transition to experience some sleep disturbances, with or without supplemental hormones. For most it passes within a year.

- Oestrogen dominance
- Excess oestrogen
- Too much caffeine
- Too much light in the bedroom

IRRITABILITY

- Low oestrogen
- Oestrogen dominance
- High testosterone
- Excess cortisol

MEMORY LOSS

- High cortisol from stress
- Low oestrogen
- Oestrogen dominance

MIGRAINES

- Oestrogen dominance

MUSCLE WEAKNESS

- Low cortisol
- Low testosterone
- Low progesterone

NIGHT SWEATS
- Low oestrogen
- Oestrogen dominance
- Low progesterone
- Fluctuating oestrogens

OSTEOPOROSIS
- Low progesterone (progesterone helps build bones)
- Low testosterone (testosterone helps build bones)
- Low oestrogen (oestrogen helps slow bone loss)
- Excess cortisol

OVARIAN CYSTS
Are often caused by too much sugar and refined carbohydrates in your diet, which raises insulin levels, thereby stimulating the ovaries to produce more androgens (male hormones).
- Oestrogen dominance

OVERSENSITIVITY
- Excess oestrogen

PAINFUL INTERCOURSE
- Low oestrogen
- Low testosterone

PMS
- Oestrogen dominance

SLEEPINESS

- Excess progesterone

SLUGGISH DIGESTION

- Excess progesterone
- Thyroid deficiency

TALKING EXCESSIVELY

- Excess oestrogen
- Excess cortisol (from stress and worrying)

THINNING SKIN

- Very high or very low cortisol
- Low testosterone
- Low oestrogen

URINARY TRACT IRRITATION AND/OR INFECTION

- Low oestrogen
- Bacterial infection
- Loss of good bacteria caused by antibiotic use

UTERINE FIBROIDS

Unknown cause, but made worse by oestrogen dominance. When they get larger, exposure to excess oestrogen or progesterone can cause them to grow.

VAGINAL DRYNESS

- Low oestrogen
- Low testosterone

WATER RETENTION, BLOATING AND/OR PUFFINESS

- Oestrogen dominance
- Excess oestrogen

WEEPINESS

- Oestrogen dominance
- Stress
- Depression

WEIGHT GAIN

- Oestrogen dominance
- Too much sugar and refined carbohydrates in your diet
- Lack of exercise
- Low thyroid

TWO REMINDERS WHEN TRACKING SYMPTOMS TO CAUSES:

- Oestrogen dominance means you do not have enough pro-gesterone to balance the effects of oestrogen. You might have oestrogen deficiency symptoms and your oestrogen might measure low, but if you have low progesterone you can still have oestrogen dominance symptoms. Your oestrogen may also be normal, but if you don't have progesterone to balance the oestrogen it will show as over production of oestrogen.

- If you are using natural hormones and find that your symptoms have returned, it's usually because:
  - You're taking a dose that is too high
  - Your timing is off.
  - You have constant overwhelming stress in your life combined with poor eating, sleeping, and exercising habits.

This chapter can be useful for both tracking your symptoms and identifying some of the causes of your symptoms. It's much easier to correct a health problem when you're aware of the underlying cause.

Now, knowing more about your symptoms and the possible causes, and which hormone levels to check, the next step is getting some answers.

CHAPTER 2

The Test with many answers

What's worse than going for a test is the fact that you don't know you need one.

The health and fitness world has been abuzz with talk about adrenal health and hormonal balance. This has left many of us looking for ways to get our hormone and adrenal levels checked out so that we can address any issues that might be standing in the way of our goals.

Hormone panel testing is normally not the first test your doctor will do so you need to take charge and request it.

Knowing what tests to do is going to set you on the road to a healthier you.

Knowing that you have certain or many of the previous chapter's symptoms and have tracked them will help you and your doctor to get you on the right treatment.

What you need to know about hormone testing and which tests to have.

Many of you are probably looking for quick, easy and affordable ways to get your hormone levels checked. Make sure that you spend your money wisely and get accurate results.

Let's talk about the best methods of evaluation to check adrenal hormones (mainly cortisol) and sex hormones like testosterone, oestrogen, and progesterone.

BLOOD TESTING OR SALIVA TESTING?

Traditionally, lab work refers to checking serum or blood levels. However, there are other methods of evaluating hormone levels such as saliva. There are pros and cons to both of these evaluation methods:

Blood testing - blood is inconvenient for many as you need to have a healthcare provider order the labs for you, you have to go to a location to have the labs drawn, and if your medical aid doesn't cover the labs, they can be quite pricey.

However, blood analysis is very accurate and tests, as well as testing facilities and labs, are highly regulated. So, with blood levels, you know you are getting reliable results.

Saliva testing - saliva or sputum tests can often be ordered by patients themselves or by non-medically licensed individuals. They are more convenient because the tests can be done at home and without scheduling an appointment, and many times the cost is not as high as blood tests. However, sputum and saliva can give you unreliable results.

Multiple studies have shown hormone levels vary significantly when salivary testing is done using cotton and polypropylene collection devices.

Cotton collection devices or "rolls" result in elevated oestradiol and testosterone levels, while polypropylene rolls result in lower oestradiol and testosterone levels.

Research has also found that small amounts of blood from the oral mucosa, variance in collection of the samples, and storage of the samples after they are collected, can cause irregularities and inaccuracy as well.

Furthermore, even if the samples are collected in the most perfect of circumstances, salivary levels of hormones vary so quickly and drastically they cannot be considered accurate. In fact, most medical aid companies will not cover the cost of these tests because of these problems.

Sputum testing for cortisol is a completely different story. Salivary cortisol measurements have been studied and are considered reliable enough to use to diagnose adrenal diseases like Cushing's syndrome.

Cortisol levels seem to be more stable and have less variance than sex hormones regardless of collection devices and storage. This is fortunate because cortisol levels should be measured at multiple times throughout the day and at night in order to assess if a person is producing appropriate amounts, at appropriate times throughout the day.

Having to send a person to a lab multiple times during a 24-hour period would be incredibly inconvenient. However, it has been proven that results of saliva cortisol tests are both reliable and consistent with serum levels and patient symptoms.

It would be incredibly convenient and easier for everyone if saliva tests were reliable enough to trust for accurate levels. But research tells us they are not as accurate as blood tests. Many patients bring in saliva tests that didn't correlate with their symptoms or their history.

WHEN SYMPTOMS DON'T MATCH THE TEST RESULTS

A female patient's saliva hormone results indicated her testosterone and oestrogen were sky-high. She was having hot flushes, low libido, wasn't sleeping, and was having drastic mood swings. Those symptoms are not consistent with high oestrogen or testosterone levels. Also, this patient was in her fifties and menopausal.

If you aren't ovulating, you probably aren't making much oestrogen or testosterone. You might be producing some testosterone from your adrenals and some oestrogen from fat cells but those levels wouldn't be clinically high. After new blood-work was done, it was discovered that her oestrogen and testosterone were actually very low.

Obtaining inaccurate saliva hormone results not only results in a waste of money, but it also prevents you from getting medical care and treatment in a timely manner.

Many people may be living with unbalanced hormones unnecessarily because their saliva tests have been incorrect. That's a big problem.

So, two things to remember:

1. Saliva for cortisol is great.
2. Blood levels for hormones like oestrogen, testosterone, progesterone and other sex hormones are your best bet.

Proper hormone balance and adrenal health is absolutely vital to your overall health and longevity, not to mention, your fitness.

HORMONE BALANCE TEST

Carefully read through the list of symptoms in each group, and put a tick next to each symptom that you have. If you tick the same symptom in more than one group, that's fine.

1. Go back and count the ticks in each group. In any group where you have two or more symptoms ticked off, there's a good chance that you have the hormone imbalance represented by that group.
2. The more symptoms that you tick off, the higher the likelihood is you have the hormone imbalance represented by that group. Some people may have more than one type of hormonal imbalance.
3. It is recommended that you print these pages and use them as a reference.
4. Go to the Women or Men's Answers Section.

HORMONE BALANCE TEST FOR WOMEN

SYMPTOM GROUP 1

PMS		Insomnia	
Early miscarriage		Painful and/or lumpy breasts	
Unexplained weight gain		Cyclical headaches	
Anxiety		Infertility	

TOTAL BOXES TICKED

If you have ticked two or more boxes in this group, go to answers to find out what type of hormonal imbalance you may have.

SYMPTOM GROUP 2

Vaginal dryness		Night sweats	
Painful intercourse		Memory problems	
Bladder infections		Lethargic depression	
Hot flushes			

TOTAL BOXES TICKED

If you have ticked two or more boxes in this group, go to answers to find out what type of hormonal imbalance you may have

SYMPTOM GROUP 3

Puffiness and bloating		Cervical dysplasia (abnormal pap smear)	
Rapid weight gain		Breast tenderness	
Mood swings		Heavy bleeding	
Anxious depression		Migraine headaches	
Insomnia		Foggy thinking	
Red flush on face		Gallbladder problems	
Weepiness			

TOTAL BOXES TICKED

If you have ticked two or more boxes in this group, go to answers to find out what type of hormonal imbalance you may have.

SYMPTOM GROUP 4

A combination of the symptoms in #1 and #3

TOTAL BOXES TICKED

If you have ticked two or more boxes in this group, go to answers to find out what type of hormonal imbalance you may have.

SYMPTOM GROUP 5

Acne		Polycystic ovary syndrome (PCOS)	
Excessive hair on the face and arms		Hypoglycaemia and/or unstable blood sugar	
Thinning hair on the head		Infertility	
Ovarian cysts		Mid-cycle pain	

TOTAL BOXES TICKED

If you have ticked two or more boxes in this group, go to answers to find out what type of hormonal imbalance you may have.

SYMPTOM GROUP 6

Debilitating fatigue		Unstable blood sugar	
Foggy thinking		Low blood pressure	
Thin and/or dry skin		Intolerance to exercise	
Brown spots on face			

TOTAL BOXES TICKED

If you have ticked two or more boxes in this group, go to answers to find out what type of hormonal imbalance you may have.

HORMONE BALANCE TEST FOR MEN

SYMPTOM GROUP 1

Weight loss		Enlarged breasts	
Loss of muscle		Lower stamina	
Lower sex drive		Softer erections	
Fatigue		Gallbladder problems	

TOTAL BOXES TICKED

If you have ticked two or more boxes in this group, go to answers to find out what type of hormonal imbalance you may have.

SYMPTOM GROUP 2

Hair loss		Headaches	
Prostate enlargement		Breast enlargement	
Irritability		Weight gain	
Puffiness/bloating			

TOTAL BOXES TICKED

If you have ticked two or more boxes in this group, go to answers to find out what type of hormonal imbalance you may have.

ANSWERS FOR WOMEN

SYMPTOM GROUP 1

Progesterone deficiency is the most common hormone imbalance among women of all ages. You may need to change your diet, get off synthetic hormones (including birth control pills), and you may need to use some progesterone cream.

SYMPTOM GROUP 2

Oestrogen deficiency is the most common hormone imbalance in menopausal women especially if you are petite and/or slim. You may need to make some special changes to your diet; take some women's herbs; and some women may even need a little bit of natural oestrogen (about one-tenth the dose prescribed by most doctors). Try saliva testing for oestradiol.

SYMPTOM GROUP 3

Excess oestrogen in women, is most often solved by getting off of the conventional synthetic hormones most often prescribed by doctors for menopausal women.

SYMPTOM GROUP 4

Oestrogen dominance is caused when you don't have enough progesterone to balance the effects of oestrogen. Thus, you can have low oestrogen but if you have even lower progesterone, you can have symptoms of oestrogen dominance. Many women between the ages of 40 and 50 suffer from oestrogen dominance. Test for progesterone and oestradiol.

SYMPTOM GROUP 5

Excess androgens (male hormones) is most often caused by too much sugar and simple carbohydrates in the diet and is often found in women who have polycystic ovary syndrome (PCOS).

SYMPTOM GROUP 6

Cortisol deficiency is caused by tired adrenals, which is usually caused by chronic stress. If you're trying to juggle a job and a family, chances are good that you have tired adrenals.

Try saliva hormone testing for the Adrenal Function or one of the individual Cortisol tests.

ANSWERS FOR MEN

SYMPTOM GROUP 1

Testosterone deficiency is most common in men over the age of fifty, and can be remedied with special nutritional supplements; increased muscle-building exercise; and supplemental hormones including (natural) testosterone, progesterone, and DHEA. It is also recommended that you get a saliva hormone test to find out which hormone(s) would be best for you. A basic set of baseline tests for men would include testosterone, DHEA, oestrogen and progesterone through a saliva test. It may also be helpful to measure morning and evening cortisol by saliva test and SHBG (Sex Hormone Binding Globulin) by blood spot test.

SYMPTOM GROUP 2

Excess oestrogen in men, can be balanced with one of the male hormones and changes in diet and lifestyle. It is also recommended that you get a saliva hormone test to pinpoint your hormone balance more exactly.

Please Note: The information contained in this Hormone Balance Test is not intended to replace a one-to-one relationship with a qualified healthcare professional, and is not intended as medical advice, but as guidelines for determining the underlying cause of your symptoms.

You are encouraged to make your healthcare decisions in partnership with a qualified healthcare professional.

CHAPTER 3

The ABC's of your hormones

WHAT ARE THESE HORMONES THAT I KEEP TELLING YOU ABOUT?

In this chapter we are going to look at each hormone, which gland it comes from, and how it functions in your body.

TYPICAL AGES THAT HORMONES DECLINE

- Age 30: human growth hormone
- Age 40: testosterone, oestrogen, progesterone
- Age 50: DHEA (a decline is noted in late 20's), thyroid hormones
- Age 60: insulin, parathyroid
- Age 70: calcitonin, erythropoietin

THESE ARE THE 20 MAIN HORMONE CULPRITS

ANDROSTENEDIONE

Androstenedione is one of the androgens/male hormones (the others being testosterone and DHEA). It is synthesised from cholesterol like all steroid hormones. Usually, when faced with male sex hormone deficiencies we concentrate on replenishing testosterone, DHEA and pregnenolone.

CALCITONIN

Calcitonin is a hormone involved in calcium metabolism and helps maintain bone. It is an often overlooked hormone that is made in your thyroid. Calcitonin loss can result in loss of bone mineral density, which can alter food choices. Frail bones, frail brain, frail body, frail life, are the associations of deteriorating musculoskeletal ageing. Musculoskeletal ageing is accelerated by growth hormone deficiency, loss of control of the parathyroid hormone, resulting in increased parathyroid hormone, decreased calcitonin and bone density loss.

Calcitonin 200 IU/d together with other hormones can be used to reverse dementia and enhance cognition.

The following hormones can enhance acetylcholine and brain cognition:

- Human growth hormone 5-90mg/month
- Vasopressin 5-60 units/d
- DHEA 5-200mg/d
- Calcitonin 200 IU/d
- Parathyroid 20-40ug/d

DHEA

DHEA is a hormone made by the adrenal glands and is the precursor of the other sex hormones. A small amount is made by the brain and skin. DHEA production declines with age, starting in the late 20s. By age 70 only about ¼ of your previous levels of DHEA are produced.

Functions of DHEA:
- Helps you deal with stress
- Supports your immune system
- Increases bone growth
- Promotes weight loss
- Decreases cholesterol and fatty deposits
- Increases brain function
- Helps your body repair itself and maintain tissues
- Decreases allergic reactions

Remember that hormones influence each other and a balanced symphony of hormones is essential. For example, insulin resistance or raised insulin influences the synthesis of testosterone and the metabolism of DHEA.

Testosterone synthesis increases and DHEA is depleted because elevated insulin increases the activity of an enzyme, 17,20–lyase, which converts more DHEA to cortisol and testosterone.

ERYTHROPOEITIN

Eryhropoeitin is produced in your kidneys and stimulates your bone marrow to make red blood cells. This is why anaemia often results when your kidneys are not functioning properly.

Eryhtropoietin supplementation at 50-100u/kg 3 times/week can increase oxygenation, reduce anaemia of renal failure, and increase red cell output of the bone marrow.

A report from the *Journal of the American Medical Association* suggests that EPO (erythropoeitin) may have a beneficial impact on congestive heart failure. It helps prevent inflammation, and studies show that it can prevent cell injury and maintain cell integrity. EPO may improve blood flow to ischemic cells starved by arterial blockages.

OESTROGENS

The body makes three main oestrogens:

- **Oestrone E1.** Many researchers believe it may be related to an increase in breast and uterine cancer.
- **Oestradiol E2.** Is the most potent oestrogen, maintaining memory, bone health and aids in protecting you from heart disease.
- **Oestriol E3.** Considerable evidence suggests that oestriol protects against breast cancer.

Oestradiol is 12 times stronger than oestrone and 80 times stronger than oestriol. High levels of oestradiol are associated with breast and uterine cancer. There are over 400 functions of oestrogen in your body.

These are the main functions of oestradiol:

- Increases HDL, lowers LDL, decreases total cholesterol, decreases triglycerides
- Decreases platelet stickiness
- Increases growth hormone
- Increases serotonin
- Increases endorphins
- Improves sleep
- Helps maintain memory
- Helps absorption of magnesium, calcium and zinc

We usually use oestradiol in varying concentrations with oestriol in a cream like Bi-est cream.

The reason we use oestrogen cream more readily than oral oestrogen is due to the following that may occur with ORAL OES-TROGEN (not with transdermal delivery):

- Increase in blood pressure
- Increase in triglycerides
- Increase oestrone E1
- Cause gallstones
- Can elevate liver enzymes
- Can decrease growth hormone (the hormone that keeps you youthful) increases SHBG (sex hormone binding globulin), can decrease testosterone
- Increases weight gain
- Increases carbohydrate craving
- Increased blood clotting factors and increased risk of thrombosis

If you are going to use oral oestrogen it is suggested to use the lowest possible dose.

For the reasons listed above, long term replenishment of oestrogen deficiency is safer using the transdermal route.

The risk/benefit ratio of replenishing oestrogen this way is superior to oral delivery. The trend is to no longer use Tri-est containing oestrone which is known to elevate cancer risk, but rather to use Bi-est in varying concentrations. But Tri-est is still used by some and is considered safer than conjugated oestrogen, progestins and synthetic oestrogens.

The following should be noted about the use of bio-identical creams:

- They are regulated by the South African Health Products Regulatory Authority (SAHPRA).
- It is not necessary to have them registered at the MCC, since registration is only required for mass production of a drug by a pharmaceutical company for mass distribution.
- Bio-identical hormone replacement is not 'one size fits all' medicine. It is an individualised, personalised, customised dosing for the particular needs of a specific patient.
- The stability of the hormones used is tested by independent laboratories.
- The efficacy is checked by assessing a patient's clinical improvement in symptoms and we can also check levels of hormones by doing the following:

- In blood tests there are limitations since these hormones are fat soluble and 'prefer' to be in the tissues than the blood. However ratios of the hormones for example oestrogen:progesterone or oestrogen:testosterone can be assessed in the bloods.
- Urine metabolite testing is readily available at laboratories like Age Diagnostic Labs (not available in SA yet, but hopefully soon will be). It is possible to send off specimens to Australia, UK, and USA for analysis.
- Saliva testing is becoming more popular abroad due to the true tissue level reflection.

- When using hormones like oestrogen it is highly recommended to assist the body to metabolise oestrogen to the healthy 2-Hydroxyestrone rather than the potentially dangerous 16 or 4-Hydroxyestrone. This can be done by supplementing with:
  - Indole-3-carbinol or DIM, daily dose recommended is 200 to 300mg
  - Moderate exercise
  - Cruciferous vegetables
  - Flax, soy, kudzu, high protein diet, omega 3, B6, B12 and folate

OESTRIOL

Considerable evidence suggests oestriol has a cancer-protective effect. Oestriol is a safer form of oestrogen with regard to breast cancer, for these reasons:

- In vitro, when given with oestradiol, oestriol accelerates the removal of oestradiol bound to protein receptors.
- Investigators have been able to initiate very little carcinogenesis in animal studies unless using extremely high doses (200-500ug/kg/day).
- Metabolism of oestriol does not result in carcinogenic substances.

Functions include:
- Menopausal symptom relief, e.g. hot flushes, insomnia, vaginal dryness
- Benefits the vaginal lining
- Helps reduce pathogenic bacteria and helps maintain healthy gut flora (lactobacilli)
- Helps restore the proper pH of the vagina
- Has been used to treat breast cancer
- Blocks oestrone by occupying the oestrogen receptor sites on breast cells
- Increases HDL (good cholesterol)

OESTRONE

This is the oestrogen made most in the postmenopausal years. High levels stimulate breast and uterine tissue and many researchers believe it may be related to an increased risk of breast cancer. Oestrone is made in your fat cells mostly in the postmenopausal years. Pre-menopausally it can be converted to oestradiol in your ovaries, but postmenopausally, little oestrone becomes oestradiol since the ovaries have stopped working. Therefore the fatter one is the more oestrone one makes. Also, alcohol consumption decreases ovarian hormone production and shifts your oestrogen production to oestrone, which increases the cancer risk.

Advantages of bio-identical oestrogens over conventional HRT:

- Topical administration versus oral has distinct advantages listed before (e.g. no increase in clotting factors resulting in potential DVT, pulmonary emboli, stroke and coronary thrombosis in elderly women).
- Bio-identical progesterone works differently to synthetic progestins. It is true that progestins have uterine/endome-trial protection, but they increase the risk for heart disease due to coronary vasospasm and increase the risk for breast cancer. Progestins also have a lot of side effects not seen with naturally produced and supplemented progesterone. (See progesterone section)
- Oestriol may protect against breast cancer.
- Bi-est transdermally is the safest way to replenish oestrogen.

- Individualised dosing is accomplished using bio-identical hormones. One size does not fit all.
- Incorporation of the hormones into a liposomal gel is a highly effective way of ensuring transdermal systemic absorption.

SOME HORMONAL AND OTHER THERAPIES FOR BREAST CANCER SURVIVORS

Oestriol is the protective oestrogen (also high during pregnancy). It does not activate the oestrogen receptor, but occupies the receptor site so that it is not available for oestradiol.

Balancing of hormones is essential and testing prior to supplementation is essential. Careful monitoring is obviously also essential.

Here are some suggestions:
- Estriol 2mg bd
- Progesterone down-regulates the oestrogen receptors in breast and uterine tissues.
- Testosterone has been reported to have an anti-carcinogenic effect on breast cancer cells and in some studies there is an increased survival rate using testosterone.
- Aromatase inhibitors like Arimidex can prevent conversion of testosterone to oestradiol and prevent conversion of androstenedione to oestrone.
- Indole-3-carbinol (I3C) prevents conversion of 2-Hydroxyestrone to the carcinogenic 16 and 4-Hydroxyestrone.

Drug therapy recommendations for high risk breast cancer patients

High risk includes previous breast cancer, two family members having breast cancer, young menarche (younger than 11), early menopause (younger than 45), obesity, and alcohol abuse.

High risk patients should consider the following:
- High dose oestriol:oestradiol supplementation (for example 90%:10%)
- Progesterone
- Indole-3-carbinol or DIM
- Melatonin
- Coenzyme Q10

HUMAN GROWTH HORMONE
Traditionally we replace growth hormone last, i.e. we first ensure all other hormone levels are normal before considering growth hormone supplementation.

Growth hormone benefits for the body:
- Cognitive benefits
- Immune function improvement
- Cardiovascular function improvement
- Improvement in body composition. As we age we lose protein/muscle mass and gain fat mass. Growth hormone reverses this since it is anabolic and lipolytic.
- Improved outcomes in traumatic brain injury
- Anti-ageing effects on the skin

There are many advantages attributed to growth hormone in adult growth hormone-deficient individuals. In fact, entire books are written on this hormone alone. We replace growth hormone by a daily subcutaneous injection. There are also secretagogues available that are a combination of amino acids which enhance your own pituitary production of growth hormone.

CORTISOL

Cortisol is the only hormone in your body that increases with age. The premature ageing that occurs with increased cortisol (a stress hormone produced by your adrenal glands, but essential for life).

Two circumstances make high levels of cortisol unhealthy:

- Long-term, chronically raised cortisol, and
- Deficiencies in cortisol's antagonistic hormones such as growth hormone, testosterone (in men), DHEA and oestradiol.

Careful avoidance of these two conditions may prevent most, if not all, ageing effects attributable to cortisol.

ALDOSTERONE

Aldosterone is a mineralocorticoid synthesised in your adrenal glands. It is essential to regulate potassium absorption in the tubules of your kidneys. Aldosterone and renin are sometimes elevated in people with elevated blood pressure. In Addison's disease, which is a non-functioning adrenal gland state, replacement of the glucocorticoids (cortisol) and the mineralocorticoids (aldosterone) are essential to maintain life. The typical picture of aldosterone deficiency or Addison's would include very low blood pressure, high potassium, low sodium, high urea, coma and even death.

INSULIN LIKE GROWTH FACTORS

Growth hormone increases IGF1 (an insulin-like growth factor in your liver). IGF1 is also a bio-identical hormone that can be administered in the same way and may be even more effective than growth hormone. Both hormones have amazing effects on weight loss, with an improvement in metabolism, appetite reduction, an increase in muscle mass, and better blood sugar regulation.

INCRETIN

Incretin is a bio-identical form of glucagon stimulation for the pancreas and blood sugar reversal. Your pancreas makes the vital hormone insulin which controls blood sugar, but two other important hormones are produced there: glucagons and somatostatin which aid in digestion and support our metabolism.

INSULIN

Insulin is the main hormone that regulates your blood sugar. If you become unresponsive to insulin (insulin resistant), your blood sugar will rise and you will develop Type 2 diabetes.

The following increase insulin levels:

- High carbohydrate diet
- Increased stress
- Decreased oestrogen
- Increased testosterone
- Insomnia
- Increased DHEA
- Decreased thyroid hormone
- Excessive progesterone
- Lack of exercise

From an anti-ageing point of view we like to have optimal youthful levels of most hormones (in other words, higher levels than post-menopausal or other pausal values).

The exceptions to this rule are: cortisol, insulin, and adrenalin. If these hormone levels are high, ageing is accelerated, so ideally we try to keep our fasting insulin levels below 5 and our stress hormones (cortisol and adrenaline) down.

MELATONIN

Melatonin is a hormone made in the pineal gland of the brain. This hormone sets your 24-hour body cycle. Melatonin is made from the amino acid tryptophan, which is also used to make serotonin. Therefore when melatonin goes up, serotonin goes down. If you eat too many high glycaemic carbohydrates you will make less melatonin and more serotonin.

Melatonin influences the following:
- Sleep
- Mood
- Stress response
- Release of sex hormones
- Antioxidant stronger than vitamin C and E
- Blocks oestrogen from binding to receptors and helps prevent cancer
- Stimulates the parathyroid gland which regulates bone formation
- Stimulates the production of growth hormone
- Decreases cortisol
- Increases the action of benzodiazepines (sleeping pills and tranquilizers).

PARATHYROID HORMONE

Bio-identical parathyroid hormone supplementation is becoming increasingly popular to treat osteoporosis. It is proven to increase spinal, hip, and total bone density over a long term period, because it mimics the body's naturally produced parathyroid hormone. In combination with other hormones like DHEA or growth hormone (if deficient) these hormones provide better bone density reversals than any of the drug therapies. Parathyroid actually activates growth hormone inside the bone and they work really well together.

PREGNENOLONE

Pregnenolone is a steroid hormone made in the adrenal glands and is the precursor to DHEA, cortisol and the sex hormones. The body synthesises this hormone from cholesterol and it is often referred to as the 'mother of all steroid hormones'. From ages 35 to 75, most people have a 65% decline in pregnenolone.

Functions:

- Increases resistance to stress
- Improves energy both physically and mentally
- Enhances nerve transmission and memory
- Reduces pain and inflammation
- Blocks the production of acid-forming compounds
- Regulates excitatory/inhibitory balance in the nervous system

Pregnenolone is used in the treatment of arthritis, depression, memory loss, fatigue, and moodiness.

PROGESTERONE

Progesterone is one of the sex hormones made in the ovaries before menopause. After menopause some progesterone is made in your adrenal glands. Progestin (synthetic progesterone) is not progesterone. Only progesterone is bio-identical.

Side effects of progestins include:

- Increased appetite
- Weight gain

- Fluid retention
- Depression
- Irritability
- Headaches
- Decreased energy
- Bloating
- Breast tenderness
- Decreased sexual interest
- Acne
- Hair loss
- Insomnia
- Breakthrough bleeding/spotting
- Stops the protective effects oestrogen has on your heart
- Increases LDL (bad cholesterol), decreases HDL (good cholesterol, protects only the uterus from cancer)
- Progestins do not prevent vasospasm (an effect opposite to progesterone)

In contrast, the following benefits are seen with progesterone – and not with progestins:

- Improved sleep
- Helps balance oestrogen
- Natural calming effect
- May protect against breast cancer
- Increases scalp hair
- Lowers cholesterol

- Lowers high blood pressure
- Helps balance fluids in cells
- Increases the beneficial effects of oestrogens on blood vessel dilation in atherosclerotic plaques
- Leaves your body much quicker than progestins, not wasting energy
- Natural antidepressant
- Increases metabolic rate
- Natural diuretic
- Has an anti-proliferative effect. Decreases the rate of cancer on all progesterone receptors, not just the uterus
- Does not change the good effect oestrogen has on blood flow

Progestins cause coronary spasm and increase the risk for heart disease. Progesterone does not.

Progesterone is a truly wonderful hormone in its natural form. It makes no sense to change its structure to a progestin and expect the same good effects. The side effects of progestins are actually progesterone deficiency.

This is because progestins bind to progesterone receptors and inhibit progesterone from binding to its receptor sites. Methods of delivery: oral micronized progesterone and transdermal cream (e.g. 3, 5 or 10% cream).

TESTOSTERONE

Androgens are often called 'male hormones'. They are testosterone, DHEA, and androstenedione. Testosterone is made in the adrenal glands and ovaries. It is important to measure both free and bound testosterone since only about 1% is free, the rest is bound to SHBG which carries the testosterone in your blood.

Testosterone has a myriad of functions in the human body:

- Motivation, emotional wellbeing, self-confidence
- Increases muscle mass and strength
- Increases sexual interest
- Helps maintain memory
- Helps maintain bone strength
- Decreases excessive body fat
- Increases muscle tone so your skin does not sag.

Ways to supplement:

Natural testosterone is the preferred method. Methyltestosterone (synthetic) has been suggested to be carcinogenic to the liver. Natural testosterone is effective as a pill or a cream.

Rotation of site of application is important to prevent hair growth.

Also remember the skin has an enzyme - aromatase, which can change the testosterone applied to oestradiol. Natural aromatase inhibitors include zinc, progesterone and chrysin.

There are natural treatments like nettle root that also increase the free testosterone from SHBG, mentioned earlier. Injectable testosterone is also available (mostly used in andropause).

THYROID HORMONES

The thyroid hormones (eltroxin/T4 and tertroxin/T3) control the rate that your body burns fuel. These two hormones are necessary in infants for the normal development of the central nervous system, in children for skeletal growth, and in adults for normal function of other organs and systems. Thyroid hormones also affect tissue growth and maturation, help regulate fat digestion, and increase intestinal absorption of carbohydrates. Typically thyropause (lowering of thyroid functioning) occurs between the ages of 30 and 40, but even more frequently at age 50.

The importance of T3, T4 and TSH (thyroid stimulating hormone from the pituitary) needs to be looked at differently to the way most doctors are taught. A partial deficiency in thyroid hormones allows life, but is a life often miserable with complaints and physical signs typical for the disease. One of the most important consequences of thyroid hormone deficiency is a decrease in the production of most other important hormones such as growth hormone, testosterone, female sex hormones, cortisol, DHEA, and others. This polyhormonal induced senescence is reversed with thyroid hormone treatment.

The best thyroid deficiency treatment should include both T4 and its more active metabolite T3.

VITAMIN D3

Yes, vitamin D3 is actually a hormone!

Vitamin D3 has numerous health benefits, over and above bone health.

According to the *Journal of Public Health*, increasing vitamin D3 intake may help lower the risk of breast cancer, colon cancer, skin cancer, prostate and ovarian cancer by as much as 50%.

Vitamin D3 has now been shown to decrease insulin resistance, regulate cell production, and modulate immune function. It also prevents and reverses skin damage. As your skin ages, it can no longer synthesise vitamin D3 from the sun. If you notice your skin is not healing the way it used to, extra vitamin D3 might be the answer.

The responsibility for your health lies with you.

It's no longer acceptable or responsible for doctors to dismiss a gradual deterioration of function and wellness as 'what happens as you get older'.

It is also not good enough to medicate symptoms as they arise, using pain relievers, antacids, arthritis drugs, and cholesterol medications. We must find a way to remain healthy, vital, and productive as we enjoy the longer lifespan that modernity has made possible.

Anti-ageing/preventative medicine will allow you to grow older without becoming aged. It will maximise your chances of not only a long life, but a long and healthy life. Anti-ageing medicine is more than just a medical speciality; it's the future of medicine and the future of humankind.

CHAPTER 4

Don't sweat the stress!

TWO MONTHS AGO, LISA, a 28-year-old mom, came to see me. She was so worn out from mothering two kids and working full-time she couldn't get out of bed. Just driving to our practice took everything she had. Her tests revealed severe adrenal imbalance and, as so often occurs in these cases, very low levels of an important hormone called DHEA.

That's why it is number three on my list of top twenty hormones.

Dehydroepiandrosterone, or DHEA, as mentioned in the previous chapter, is a steroid hormone synthesised from cholesterol and secreted by the adrenal glands. The adrenals are walnut-sized organs located right above your kidneys. The average adult makes about 25 mg of DHEA per day (some more, some less) with dwindling production as we get older. Men at all ages have more DHEA than women.

DHEA production is at its highest in your twenties: by the time we reach seventy we only make about 20% of the DHEA we had when we were young. A decline in DHEA with the passage of time is clearly what nature intended and as far as we know, is a healthy process.

This is only one of the major reasons we don't recommend self-prescribing DHEA through over-the-counter products.

The body uses DHEA to make androgens and oestrogens, the male and female sex hormones. DHEA is an adrenal steroid hormone in the body. It is made by the adrenal glands and is then converted to androgens, estrogens and other hormones. These are the hormones that regulate fat and mineral metabolism, sexual and reproductive function, and energy levels.

DHEA is known to be a precursor, to the numerous steroid hormones, including oestrogen and testosterone, which serve well known functions, but the specific biological role of DHEA itself is not so well understood. It is difficult for researchers to separate the effects of DHEA from those of the primary sex steroids into which it is metabolised.

Although the specific mechanisms of action of DHEA are only partly understood, supplemental

DHEA has been shown to have anti-ageing, anti-obesity, and anti-cancer influences. In addition, it is known to stabilise nerve cell growth and is being tested in Alzheimer's patients.

Another reason is that DHEA is a very powerful precursor to all of your major sex hormones: oestrogen, progesterone, and testosterone (its molecular structure is closely related to testosterone). We call it the "mother hormone" — the source that fuels the body's metabolic pathway.

Besides DHEA, your adrenals also make the stress hormones cortisol and adrenaline. Adrenal exhaustion from coping with chronic stress — from (among other things) poor nutrition, yo-yo dieting, emotional turmoil, and job-related stress — means your adrenals are bone-tired from pumping out cortisol and they simply can't manufacture enough DHEA to support a healthy hormonal balance. The end result is that you feel tapped out, overwhelmed and, often, depressed.

It's likely that DHEA and adrenal function are related to neuro-transmitter-release rates based on the mood elevation our patients report after just two weeks of adrenal support. But more research is needed to isolate the individual effects of DHEA from the hormones it gets metabolised into before we can know for sure what part it plays in all of this.

One thing we do know is that adequate levels of DHEA are needed to ensure your body can produce the hormones it needs when it needs them. In that balanced state your mood is stable and you feel clear-headed, joyful and vigorous. DHEA is the best 'feel-good' hormone we know. And it works quickly and effectively when taken with the right combination of support.

When DHEA levels are low, your body does not have enough working material for proper endocrine function. This throws off your hormone production and you feel a general sense of malaise, along with other symptoms of hormonal imbalance — how severe depends on how many other demands are being made on your body at the same time.

There is a growing body of evidence that healthy levels of DHEA may help stave off Alzheimer's disease, cancer, osteoporosis, depression, heart disease and obesity, but there is still no clear-cut consensus. There may be some increased risks associated with DHEA for women with a history of breast cancer — all the more reason to take DHEA under medical supervision.

In my practice I use DHEA where I've seen reliable proof of efficacy — in cases of adrenal and other hormone imbalance.

DHEA AND ADRENAL IMBALANCE

Your lifestyle, diet, and stress levels all contribute to the amount of DHEA your body can produce in a given period. In my practice I look first and foremost at adrenal function, using DHEA levels as one of several diagnostic tools.

Think of our exhausted mother, Lisa. Like her, your adrenals work tirelessly to meet the demands placed on them until they are utterly exhausted. Without adequate support, they spiral downward into adrenal imbalance and eventually adrenal fatigue.

Most of the patients I see at my practice — and I mean 99% — have some indication of adrenal imbalance, including symptoms of low DHEA levels such as: depression, women problems, general health issues, and extreme adrenal fatigue.

These result in:

- Decrease in muscle mass
- Decrease in bone density
- Depression
- Aching joints
- Loss of libido
- Lowered immunity

Sounds a lot like hormone imbalance!

Stress is the number one cause of most diseases we experience today and the number one cause of death.

We all live under huge amounts of stress every day, some good, but mostly bad. The only way to keep your body in a healthy balance is to learn to deal with stress and to limit it.

PART THREE

YOUR HORMONE SOLUTION AND PLAN

Your illness does not define you…
Your strength and courage does!

CHAPTER 1

Bio-identical Hormone Replacement Therapy (BHRT) vs. Non-identical

O PTIMISING THE WONDERFUL SYMPHONY of bio-identical hormones is key to optimal health – along with good nutrition, good lifestyle choices and moderate exercise.

Mother Nature gave us these hormones and for many centuries they have withstood many challenges and the human race has survived. We cannot change the structure of nature's hormones and expect the same effects.

In fact, we often see very harmful effects. Countless studies show worse outcomes when the structure of a hormone is changed. Bio-identical replacement is all about the use of the structurally identical hormones found in your body.

Supplementing with bio-identical hormones as we age, to more youthful levels of hormones, may retard the degenerative processes that occur with the ageing process.

It is becoming increasingly accepted that we age prematurely because our hormone levels decline, and that if we restore hormone levels to the optimal range we avoid many of the ageing diseases. Hormone deficiency has been linked to diseases like cancer, heart disease, diabetes mellitus, dementia, osteoporosis, and osteoarthritis.

Other consequences include visual and hearing loss, fractures, frailty, incontinence, obesity, reduced libido, and degenerative neurological diseases. Additionally, hormone deficiency can cause cancer, such as the low testosterone levels associated with prostate cancer or the low levels of progesterone involved in breast cancer.

In the early days of the controversial *Women's Health Initiative* (WHI) studies, new results confirmed the health risks of long-term use of combination (oestrogen plus progestin) hormone therapy in healthy, postmenopausal women persist even years after stopping the drugs and clearly outweigh the benefits.

Researchers report that about three years after women stopped taking combination hormone therapy, many of the health effects of hormones such as increased risk of heart disease are diminished, but overall risks, including risks of stroke, blood clots, and cancer, remain high. The WHI is sponsored by the National Heart, Lung, and Blood Institute (NHLBI) of the National Institutes of Health (NIH).

It is crucial to differentiate between toxic and safe hormone replenishment. Bio-identical hormone replenishment is a powerful protective agent against serious diseases. Understanding the difference between bio-identical and non-bio-identical hormones can greatly enhance your quality of life.

Why synthetic, non-bio-identical hormones have so many side effects

Synthetic and pharmaceutical hormones are artificial chemicals that attempt to replicate human hormones. They are structurally foreign to the body. While bio-identical hormones have the identical molecular structure to human hormones, enabling easy metabolism, synthetic hormones are altered to have a different chemical make-up than natural hormones. It is this structural difference that has caused so many side effects over the years in HRT.

The immune system is well-documented to attack anything it perceives as foreign or toxic to the body. From an evolutionary aspect, it takes millennia to become accustomed to a new chemical entity. New foreign chemical entities are fraught with dangers, even in our food.

An example is the relatively recent hydrogenation of liquid plant oils into foreign saturated fats and the formation of transfats in food production. These foreign fats have only been around for the last 50 years and they result in increases in heart disease and cancer. Conversely, unsaturated plant oils reduce the risk of heart disease and cancer (e.g. olive oil, flaxseed oil and coconut oil – all rich in omega 3 fats).

Similarly, synthetic non-bio-identical hormones have been around for less than 50 years, compared to bio-identical ones, which have existed in our bodies since the birth of the human race. These synthetic hormones are associated with increased side effects and can very often be detrimental to your health. If they are used at inappropriate doses and for too long a time period or in ageing people who have diseased blood vessels, there may be an associated increased risk for very serious medical complications. These complications include breast cancer or thrombotic disorders like deep vein thrombosis, stroke or heart attack. This is made worse if the hormones are administered orally, since the oral route greatly increases the production of blood clotting factors, via the first pass liver effect. This first pass metabolism does not occur with the transdermal route, and so blood clotting risk and thrombosis is reduced this way.

Pharmaceutical hormones like diethylstilbestrol, methyl testosterone, conjugated oestrogens, medroxyprogesterones and birth control pills have all been linked to cancer.

In recent years, several studies showed that women taking HRT have a higher risk of breast cancer, heart disease, stroke, and blood clots. The largest study was the Women's Health Initiative (WHI), a 15-year study tracking over 161 800 healthy, postmenopausal women. The study found that women who took the combination therapy had an increased risk of heart disease. The overall risks of long-term use outweighed the benefits, the study showed.

But after that, a handful of studies based on WHI research have focused on the type of therapy, the way it's taken, and when treatment started. Those factors can produce different results. One recent study by the Fred Hutchinson Cancer Research Centre reveals that antidepressants offer benefits similar to low-dose oestrogen without the risks.

With all the conflicting research, it's easy to see why HRT can be confusing.

Who shouldn't take Hormone Replacement Therapy?

If you have these conditions, you may want to avoid HRT:

- Blood clots
- Cancer (such as breast, uterine, or endometrial)
- Heart or liver disease
- Heart attack
- Known or suspected pregnancy
- Stroke
- What are the side effects of Hormone Replacement Therapy?
- HRT comes with side effects such as:
- Bloating
- Breast swelling or tenderness
- Headaches
- Mood changes
- Nausea
- Vaginal bleeding
- Osteoporosis
- Breast cancer
- Heart disease
- Type 2 diabetes

WHY BIO-IDENTICAL HORMONES ARE RECOMMENDED

In the 1960s Dr Charles Huggins received a Nobel Prize for his work with bio-identical hormones by decreasing the size of cancer tumours. But his work has been overlooked for decades. Today it's concluded there are great risks in prescribing synthetic HRT, bio-identical hormones are clearly the safest option.

Bio-identical hormones are entirely the same as human hormones.

The chemical structure is the same as that produced naturally in the human body. Bio-identical hormone replenishment is used to restore hormone levels to normal physiological levels, based on blood tests; not at supra-physiological mega doses, based on symptoms alone as is often the case with non-bio-identical, synthetic hormones. As mentioned previously, these hormones are mostly administered transdermally to avoid first pass metabolism in the liver.

Bio-identical hormones are an integral part of maintaining health and a tremendous anti-ageing tool. Bio-identical hormones have been used in Europe and America for over 15 years and are a lot safer, have fewer side effects, and are not linked to cancer at all.

THE BENEFITS OF PHARMACY COMPOUNDING OF INDIVIDUALISED MEDICINES

Compounded medicines are unique, individualised pharmaceutical products formulated and adjusted to a patient's specific needs, symptoms or blood results. They allow for flexible dosages, concentrations, combinations and numbers of actives to be incorporated into one product.

Pharmacy compounding has been an essential part of healthcare since the earliest days of pharmacy. It is always prescribed by a physician or doctor in order to meet the needs of patients. As a valued part of today's healthcare, compounding currently supplies intravenous mixtures, parenteral nutrition solutions, paediatric preparations, and pain-management medications for patients whose medical needs would otherwise go unmet.

The following factors continue to influence doctors and their prescribing habits:

- We cannot always believe information provided by the media which most often reflects the goals of advertisers.
- Consider the money trail (e.g. industry and managed care).
- Citizen response does make a difference.
- The pharmaceutical industry spends huge amounts of money on marketing of patentable non-bio-identical hormones. Bio-identical hormones are not patentable, and so not profitable for pharmaceutical companies to develop and market.

NATURAL OR BIO-IDENTICAL HORMONES

Hormones are called natural or bio-identical if they are an exact duplicate of what your body makes. In other words, the molecular structure of a natural hormone is identical to that of the hormones made by your body. This is an important distinction because the hormones typically handed out by your doctor are not natural. Some of them are completely man-made and are found nowhere in nature and others notably Premarin is made from the urine of pregnant mares.

According to the most recent census data there are about 37.5 million women (ages 40 to 59) reaching or currently at menopause. For many consumers, 'natural' implies 'safer'. That perception explains the demand for natural products.

Often however, the manufacturing of natural products is not well-regulated and the significance of the word 'natural' has different meanings for consumers and manufacturers.

Natural hormone replacement therapy (NHRT) is a misnomer. Bio-identical hormone replacement therapy (BHRT) is the proper term.

BIO-IDENTICAL HORMONE REPLACEMENT THERAPY

As mentioned, bio-identical hormones have the exact molecular structure as those made in the human body. In other words, the two are indistinguishable from each other. Bio-identical hormones produce the same physiological responses as those of endogenous hormones (the body's natural hormones).

The Food and Drug Administration (FDA) considers bio-identical hormones to be natural regardless of their source, and as a result, they cannot be patented.

MISCONCEPTIONS ABOUT BIO-IDENTICAL HORMONES

Many people are unfamiliar with the significance of bio-identical hormones. It seems they are more concerned about the source of the hormones rather than the effects produced by those hormones. Bio-identical hormones can be extracted and derived from a variety of different sources such as plants (soy or sweet potato) or animals (pigs or horses). They can also be produced synthetically. However, hormones of plant or animal extraction that are bio-identical to human hormones are still not completely natural in the purest sense, because they undergo a laboratory process and several processing steps before the bio-identical end-product is obtained.

THE IMPORTANT ISSUES WHEN DECIDING BIO-IDENTICAL THERAPY

Natural hormone replacement therapy involves two important issues - the source of the product trying to acquire a natural source from plants, and the end-product trying to obtain something bio-identical. Which is more important?

The physiological effect, of a bio-identical product should be the most important focus. Women are most comfortable with hormones that are obtained from a plant source and are seen as bio-identical. Few commercially available products fit this description. But, thanks to the WHI findings that exposed the failure of synthetic hormone replacement, women are selecting what has been available for over 20 years, bio-identical hormones that are plant derived.

A pharmaceutical company's profits come from patents that ensure them that no other company can manufacture a product like theirs for seven years. Hence, the cost of this product is determined entirely by them.

There are several new products that have been marketed as being natural because they are derived from plants such as soy or sweet potatoes, but few are truly natural because they are not

bio-identical. Sometimes, a bio-identical hormone is combined with another completely synthetic non-bio-identical hormone and the results are advertised as a natural product.

Premarin for example is advertised as a natural oestrogen replacement therapy because it is derived from the urine of a pregnant mare, but it is not bio-identical to human oestrogen and has been found to have devastating effects on women. The manufacturer of this product is beginning to prepare for the national class action suit for the greatest hoax on women in the last century. The benefits that they claimed women would receive were not only false; their drug actually ended countless women's lives.

BIO-IDENTICAL HORMONES- NATURONE NATURAL PROGESTERONE

Integrative pharmaceuticals use natural plant compounds to create the bio-identical hormone progesterone. The percentage used is 1.6% or 20mg per dispensing transdermal dose. 20 mg has been found to be the appropriate dose for women needing to supplement with progesterone. Naturone can be purchased in South Africa.

The following information on commercially compounded and natural hormone replacement products is featured. The source of the ingredients is listed and whether it is considered bio-identical.

BIO-IDENTICAL OESTROGEN
- Micronized oestradiol / Estrace – synthesised from soy and sweet potato
- Oestradiol / Alora - synthetic
- Oestradiol / Climara - synthesised from soybeans
- Oestradiol / Estraderm - synthesised from sweet potato
- Oestradiol / Fem Patch - synthetic
- Oestradiol / Vivelle, Vivelle-Dot - synthesised from sweet potato
- Oestradiol / Estring - synthesised from sweet potato

NON-BIO-IDENTICAL OESTROGEN

- Conjugated oestrogens / Premarin - pregnant mares' urine
- Conjugated oestrogens / Cenestin - synthesised from soy and sweet potato
- Esterified oestrogens (oestrone, equilin) / Estra Tab - both oestrone and equillin are synthesised from soy and sweet potato
- Esterified oestrogens (oestrone, equillin) / Menest- both oestrone and equillin are synthesised from soy and sweet potato
- Estropipate / Ogen - synthesised from sweet potato
- Estropipate / Ortho-Est - synthesised from sweet potato
- Ethinylestradiol / Estinyl - synthesised from sweet potato
- Estradiol cypionate / Depo–Estradiol - synthetic
- Estradiol valerate / Deloestrogen - synthetic

Use phyto-oestrogens not oestrogens

A phyto-oestrogen is a naturally-occurring plant nutrient that exerts an oestrogen-like action on the body without the harmful effects of oestrogen. This is what the Japanese women have used and why they have almost a non-existent occurrence of menopause symptoms and a greatly reduced cancer rate compared to the United States. It is believed that the xenohormone exposure that exists in the U.S. creates endocrine disruption. Xenohormones are any substance that acts on the endocrine system/hormone production to exert an outside influence on receptor cells, and therefore, hormone receptors throughout the body.

Many women experience oestrogen dominance, a condition where a woman can have deficient, normal or excessive oestrogen, but has little or no progesterone to balance its effects in the body. Even a woman with low oestrogen levels can have oestrogen dominance symptoms if she doesn't have enough progesterone.

Phyto-oestrogens bind to oestrogen receptor sites preventing too much oestrogen and thereby rebalancing the hormones. Phyto-oestrogens are identifiable to your body; they are easily cleaved from your oestrogen receptor sites and stimulate them for a short time.

Synthetic forms of oestrogen are unidentifiable and your body does not possess the enzymes to cleave or separate them from our receptor sites. This results in excess stimulation of endocrine tissues; breast, uterus, and ovaries. If we look at the body closely we find that all tissue; hair, skin, mucous membranes/vaginal tissue, subcutaneous fat, and even the brain tissue is adversely affected by excess synthetic oestrogens found in your environment. All petrochemical derived products exert an oestrogen-like influence on your body. Petrochemical derived products; all pharmaceutical drugs, plastic, Styrofoam, herbicides, pesticides... the list is frightening.

BIO-IDENTICAL PROGESTERONE

- Micronized progesterone / Promethium - synthesised from sweet potato
- Micronized progesterone / Crinone - synthesised from sweet potato
- Micronized progesterone - synthesised from Non-GMO sweet potato

NON-BIO-IDENTICAL PROGESTERONE

- Medroxyprogesterone acetate / Provera - synthetic
- Medroxyprogesterone acetate / Cycrin - synthetic
- Medroxyprogesterone acetate / Amen - synthetic

BIO-IDENTICAL PROGESTERONE FOR MENOPAUSAL WOMEN

Research reveals that the traditional treatment methods for menopause were wrong. Synthetic hormone replacement therapy is very harmful and much less effective than bio-identical progesterone. Research unearthed that bio-identical progesterone not only eliminates many or most menopausal symptoms, it effectively negates the harmful side effects of synthetic hormones.

COMBINATION HRT (TWO OR MORE HORMONES), NON-BIO-IDENTICAL

- Conjugated oestrogens and Medroxy progesterone acetate / PremPro-Pregnant mares' urine - synthetic
- Conjugated oestrogens and Medroxy progesterone acetate/ PremPhase-Pregnant mares' urine - synthetic
- Esterified oestrogens and Methyltestosterone acetate/EstraTest HS - synthesised from soy and sweet potato
- Esterified oestrogens and Methyltestosterone acetate/Estra Test -synthesised from soy and sweet potato and a synthetic
- Ethinyl estradiol and Norethindrone acetate/Femhrt - synthesised from soy
- Oestradiol and Norgestinate /OrthoPrefest - synthesised from soy and a synthetic

- Oestradiol and Norethindrone acetate /Combipatch - synthesised from soy and synthesised from sweet potato
- Oestradiol and Norethindrone acetate/Activella - synthetic

COMPOUNDED HORMONE REPLACEMENT THERAPY, BIO-IDENTICAL

Formulated by a specialising compounding pharmacy and individually mixed for each woman based on a profile that is done by her blood. A saliva test is preferable as it is more accurate.

- Oestrone, Oestradiol and Oestriol (triple oestrogen)/compounded - synthesised from soy
- Oestradiol and Oestriol (bi-oestrogen)/compounded - synthesised from soy
- Oestriol / compounded - synthesised from soy
- Progesterone cream-Progensa 20

Bio-identical progesterone reduces the symptoms and discomfort of menopause, premenopause, and PMS without the side effects associated with synthetic hormone replacement therapy.

PROGESTERONE PLUS WITH PHYTOESTROGENS

Bio-identical progesterone with phytoestrogens will reduce the symptoms and discomfort of menopause, perimenopause, and premenstrual syndrome without the side effects associated with synthetic hormone replacement therapy.

CHAPTER 2

Longevity with BHRT

T HE FOLLOWING ARE A few of the benefits that can be obtained with bio-identical hormone replacement therapy enhancing health, happiness, and vitality through anti-ageing.

Benefits of bio-identical hormone therapy for men and women include:

Balanced moods: Hormone fluctuations can cause mood swings due to hormonal interference with blood sugar and brain chemistry. Balanced hormones can remedy feelings of anger, anxiety, and depression.

Increased muscle mass: A testosterone deficiency can occur in both men and women.

Testosterone directly affects the building of muscle. If testosterone levels are too low muscle mass will decrease.

Fat loss: Muscle influences the burning of calories. When muscle is abundant, fat stores are tapped into in order to sustain energy. If oestrogen is low for either a man or woman, the body attempts to conserve oestrogen by storing extra fat. This is because fat contains oestrogen.

Adding regular amounts of oestrogen to the body can decrease fat storage.

Higher libido: If hormone levels are decreased, then desire for sexual activity is also decreased. When hormones are restored to normal levels, libido is boosted.

Healthier sleeping patterns: The body's internal clock sets sleeping patterns and is located in the part of the brain known as the hypothalamus. Hormonal imbalances can interfere with signals in the hypothalamus and create disturbed sleep.

Increased vitality: Fluctuations of hormones can cause blood sugar to not be processed properly, and this can cause feelings of fatigue. When hormones are balanced, the body can effectively produce energy to restore and increase vitality.

Higher bone density: Oestrogen and testosterone influence the way bones absorb calcium.

If the bones cannot properly absorb calcium, they become weak, which leads to osteoporosis.

Balanced hormones can regulate calcium absorption to keep bones healthy and strong.

Decreased hot flushes: The hypothalamus is the body's internal thermometer. Hormonal deficiencies can cause signals going to the hypothalamus to get crossed, and this can result in hot flushes and night sweats.

Increased vaginal lubrication: Vaginal tissue needs oestrogen to be healthy. Low oestrogen levels can cause vaginal dryness. By supplementing the deficient hormones, vaginal dryness can be relieved.

Increased skin elasticity: Collagen is responsible for skin youth and elasticity. When the collagen bonds break apart, skin can appear dry or wrinkled. Vitamin C and oestrogen influence the formation of collagen and help keep skin youthful.

Improved erectile function: Testosterone directly affects reproductive functions. Sexual functions may be decreased when testosterone is deficient and improved when testosterone levels are brought back to normal.

Reduced hair thinning: Testosterone assists hair follicles in the producing of hair, and cells can die away due to a lack of hormonal production and dryness.

Restored muscle mass: When testosterone levels decline, men can lose between five to seven kilograms of lean muscle mass. Restoring testosterone to healthy levels improves the ability of muscles to regenerate with exercise.

The debate and discussion over the safety of Hormone Replacement Therapy continues to remain a focal issue in anti-ageing medicine.

In 2002 in the United States, the National Heart, Lung, and Blood Institute (NHLBI), a government agency, stopped the large-scale, multi-centre trial of combined oestrogen and progestin therapy, administered as part of the group's WHI study of healthy menopausal women.

The researchers terminated this study element because they found an increased risk of invasive breast cancer and coronary heart disease that outweighed the benefits from the hormone replacement therapy.

However, NHLBI failed to disclose that their researchers did not use bio-identical hormones in the treatment. Bio-identical hormones have the same chemical structure as hormones that are made in the human body.

As mentioned, the term 'bio-identical' indicates that the chemical structure of the replacement hormone is identical to that of the hormone naturally found in the human body. In order for a replacement hormone to fully replicate the function of hormones which were originally naturally produced and present in the human body, the chemical structure must exactly match the original.

Bio-identical replacement therapy (BHRT) is a method by which replaced hormones follow normal metabolic pathways so that the essential active metabolites are formed in response to the treatment. The molecular differences between bio-identical and non-bio-identical hormones may prove to be the defining aspect in terms of HRT safety, and failure to make this differentiation and thereby alarm the public could be construed as misleading.

Natural rather than synthetic forms of hormones are associated with greater bio-availability, as they are taken up by the body more readily and utilised more effectively.

Safe optimisation of essential hormone levels for you, if deficient and symptomatic, is the goal of anti-ageing endocrinology. This requires careful monitoring of bio-available hormone levels.

This also requires establishment of baseline laboratory data and regular analysis on at least a semi-annual basis in order to achieve the safest and most effective hormonal balance at the lowest possible dose.

The goal of BHRT is to optimise function and prevent morbidity with ageing, and to enhance quality of life. With proper modification, adjustment, and titration by an experienced anti-ageing physician, the benefits of BHRT far outweigh the risks. Anti-ageing physicians remain steadfastly at the helm advancing bio-identical hormone replacement therapy, thereby providing crucial research data ultimately to negate the controversy and confirm the safety and efficacy of BHRT.

CHAPTER 3

Anti-ageing:
the hormone tightrope

A s a result of declining fertility and increasing longevity, the populations of a growing number of countries are aging rapidly. Between 2005 and 2050, half of the increase in the world population will be accounted for by a rise in the population aged 60 years or over, whereas the number of children (persons under age 15) will decline slightly. Furthermore, in the more developed regions, the population aged 60 or over is expected to nearly double (from 245 million in 2005 to 406 million in 2050), whereas that of persons under age 60 will probably decline (from 971 million in 2005 to 839 million in 2050).

As one ages, changes occur in all body systems including the endocrine system. These changes may be due to the amount of hormones secreted or the sensitivity of target organs. In some cases, the changes in amount of hormones secreted may be secondary to changes in target organs (e.g. LH and FSH). In addition, there may also be some change in the rate of metabolism of other hormones (e.g. increased peripheral degradation of thyroid hormones).

Hormones, with their power to roll back the effects of ageing and boost sexual activity, have always been regarded with a mixture of fascination and alarm.

In the first half of the last century, before testosterone or oestrogen were synthesised, there were lurid accounts of wealthy elderly males practising an adventurous and eye-watering form of anti-ageing medicine by grafting the crushed testicles of chimpanzees and other mammals onto their own which, they claimed, was hugely rejuvenating.

Much more concern and confusion now centres on HRT, which is composed of synthetic versions of the 'female' hormones, oestrogen and progesterone. The apparent panacea turned out to have a dark side, when HRT was found to actually raise the risk of heart disease and breast cancer following the WHI study in 2002. This has left millions of women in their forties and fifties in a dilemma. Do you plump for the benefits of HRT and hope to avoid the side effects? Or do you stay off it and hope to find something else? Official medical advice is that short-term use – two years – is not linked with any added risks. Even so, many have stopped taking it. In the wake of the 2002 study, the number of prescriptions in the UK and the US has halved. In the years since there has also been a significant decline in the number of breast cancers.

NATURAL VS. SYNTHETIC HORMONES

The ones used in HRT are not identical, and this is very probably the reason for the problems they have caused; for example, a type of oestrogen still widely used (over 500 000 prescriptions were issued in

England alone in 2010) is known as conjugated oestrogen and comes from the urine of pregnant mares, so it contains types of oestrogen normally only found in horses. The best-known brand is Premarin, and this was used in the WHI trial.

The replacement for progesterone that is used in regular HRT is known as progestin (or progestagen), and the best-known brand is Provera. It also has a significantly different chemical structure from progesterone.

This is linked to the very different effects the two have:

- Progesterone is the hormone made in large amounts during pregnancy, it is also a diuretic, and it decreases the risk of blood clots, has antidepressant effects and helps to build bone.
- Progestins can cause miscarriages, fluid retention and blood clots, and are linked with mood swings and can reduce bone density.

HORMONES DECLINE WITH AGE

The fact is that hormone levels do often decline dramatically later in life. Testosterone deficiency can result in lack of sex drive, lack of motivation, and depression in both men and women. Lack of oestrogen results in vaginal dryness and lack of progesterone, from which all these hormones can be made, results in lack of everything. Also, progesterone dampens down adrenal hormones so a common effect of progesterone deficiency is more anxiety, bursts of anger, insomnia and tight and aching muscles, all of which are often found during menopause.

As you can see from the diagram below progesterone is the 'mother' of all hormones, and is made from cholesterol. (Beware statin enthusiasts – driving down cholesterol too low e.g. below 3.5mmol/l could lead to hormone deficiency.)

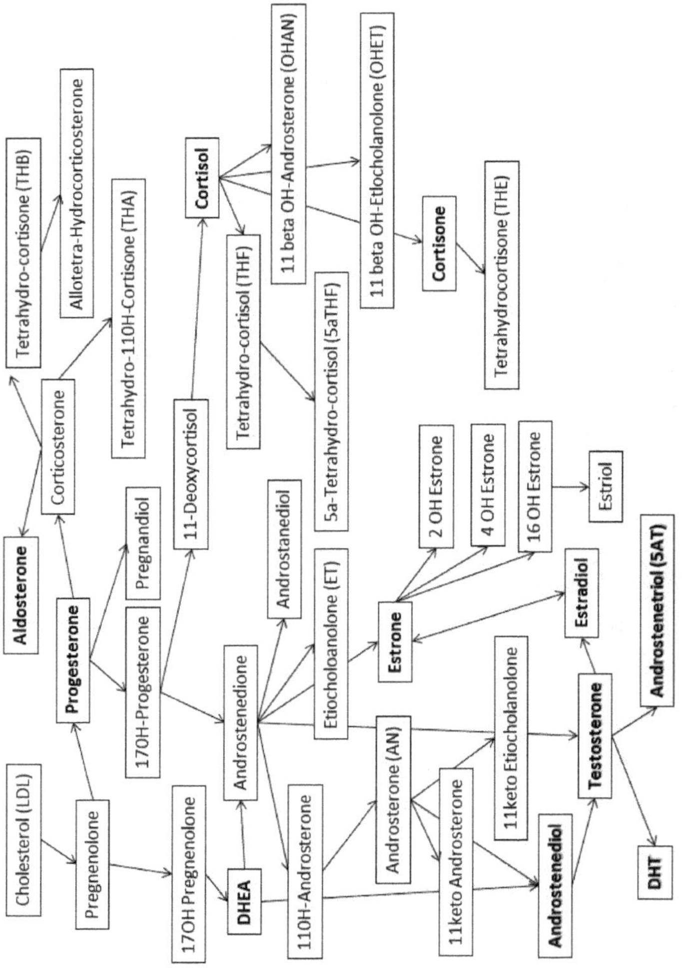

The Hormone Cascade

The body will always make cortisol – the stress hormone – in prefer-
ence to anything else because it is to do with our immediate survival.
This may not actually be the case when you get stressed watching
the news but your body thinks it is. Consequently, DHEA levels
drop. The more stressed you are the higher the cortisol and the
lower the DHEA, until you are completely burnt out in which case
both drop significantly. This in turn means that there is less DHEA
to manufacture testosterone. Chronically low amounts of DHEA
is one of the consistent indicators that you are ageing faster than
your chronological age, which is why it has become such a popular
supplement.

DHEA – DO YOU NEED IT?

DHEA is the most abundant hormone in the body, but production
for both men and women peaks at age 20 and it is reduced to half that
rate by age 40, and by the time you are 65 you will only be producing
10–20 per cent of your youthful level. It's part of the pathway that
produces the sex hormones so it is likely to have an impact there and
it is also the hormone that balances cortisol, the stress hormone. This
means that low levels can reduce the effectiveness of the immune
system, which becomes less responsive when you're stressed.

So there is certainly a logical case for restoring your levels. DHEA
supplements benefit mice, but there is not yet any hard proof that
they slow down ageing in humans.

Symptoms of a deficiency include:

- Feeling burnt out
- Unable to cope with stress
- Insomnia
- Lack of drive or motivation

Your body naturally produces 35–60mg of DHEA a day, which can be accurately measured in both saliva and blood. Practitioners are likely to prescribe between 15mg and 50mg. If you are taking DHEA, you should re-check your level after about 90 days. I sometimes recommend it to people who are burnt out for one month only, at a dose of 25mg.

The other way to increase your DHEA level is to reduce your stress and so bring down your cortisol level. Some very simple exercises you can do that have been being shown to be helpful:

- Yoga
- Weight lifting and resistance training
- Breathing techniques like in Tai Chi
- Meditation
- Walking

These exercises have been found to eliminate negative thought loops and to promote sustained positive emotional states. In one study with 45 volunteers, the 15 who did the exercises for a month saw their cortisol drop by 23 % and their DHEA level increase by 100 %. They also reported feeling much less stressed and more positive. There was no change in the others.

TO PROGESTERONE OR NOT TO PROGESTERONE

Many hormone experts think that all post-menopausal women should be on physiological levels of progesterone, because none is produced by the ovaries after menopause and your body uses it to make other hormones.

It is needed to protect your bones: stimulating the bone-building osteoblasts while oestrogen damps down the demolition team of the osteoclasts. In fact, it could be that progesterone plays a larger role in bone protection than oestrogen. Women who have periods when no progesterone is produced – known as anovulatory – start to lose bone mass; however, the results from trials using progesterone to protect bones have been contradictory; for example, one found that it was four times more effective than oestrogen HRT, with none of the associated risks, whereas two more found no effect, although menopausal symptoms, such as hot flushes and night sweats, were reduced.

Could you be deficient? These are the symptoms to watch out for:

- Anxiety, depression, irritability and mood swings
- Loss of bone mass/increased risk of osteoporosis
- Increased pain and inflammation
- Insomnia
- Decreased HDL cholesterol
- Excessive menstruation

If you have two or more positive answers you could well benefit from seeing an expert.

How can you be certain that you won't be at the same risk of cancer as women taking HRT?

You can't be absolutely certain, but there is evidence that combining oestrogen with progesterone is considerably safer than the progestin– oestrogen combination. Randomised trials haven't been done, but there is a very interesting natural experiment underway in France where both progestins and progesterone are widely used, because some women prefer one and some the other.

Researchers have followed over 80 000 women to see what happens to those in each group, and the result was a convincing win for progesterone, which caused no increase in cancer.

Those getting the progestin combination, however, had their risk raised by 69%. Taking oestrogen alone raised the risk by 29%.

The licensed oral progesterone used in France is called Utrogestan. Doctors can also prescribe

Pro-juven, a transdermal progesterone cream, as an unlicensed medicine.

OESTROGENS

During middle age, a woman's level of the three oestrogen hormones begins to decline, because these hormones are no longer needed to prepare the womb lining for pregnancy.

One effect of this is that menstrual flow becomes lighter and often irregular, until eventually it stops altogether.

Other signs of declining level of oestrogen include:

- Thinner, older skin with more wrinkles
- Vaginal dryness
- Increased risk of urinary tract infections
- Decreased sex drive
- Loss of bone mass

Once again, if these seem familiar, you could benefit from being checked out. Even if your oestrogen level is low, you could still be suffering from oestrogen dominance.

Symptoms of which include:

- Water retention
- Breast tenderness
- Mood swings
- Weight gain around the hips and thighs
- Depression
- Loss of libido
- Cravings for sweets

This seems counterintuitive, but it's because oestrogen and progesterone need to be kept in balance. So if you are in your forties and having anovulatory periods, you could be in a state of oestrogen dominance, even though your oestrogen is low, because your progesterone levels are even lower.

The result can be too many growth signals to the cells of the breast and womb, raising the risk of cancer. This is why you need a good practitioner. Just replacing low oestrogen without checking what else is going on might not make you feel better and could lead to cancer.

To complicate matters further, you don't just replace 'oestrogen'. It comes in three varieties –

- Oestrodial
- Oestrone
- Oestriol

Furthermore, they are present in very different proportions.

Oestriol is the weakest and pre-menopausal women normally have lots of it; it makes up about 90% of the total amount. The next most abundant is oestradiol, the most potent one, at around 7%, followed by oestrone at 3%.

Bio-identical practitioners will test to find the proportions of your oestrogens and then prescribe accordingly. 'I often find that oestrone levels are elevated in post-menopausal women, while oestradiol and oestriol are too low.' More than half my patients are prescribed progesterone along with a combination of bio-identical oestradiol and oestriol.

TESTOSTERONE

Although testosterone is also present in women, it is men who experience most of the problems when levels are low. In women it is strongly linked to lack of sex drive and often given in small doses by bio-identical hormone practitioners.

Just as the decline of oestrogen and progesterone lead to many of the key signs of female ageing, falling testosterone does the same for men. In both cases there is a decline in sexuality, along with thinning bones, thickening waists, fading memory, emotional swings, aching joints, and night sweats.

According to Dr Malcolm Carruthers, who has compiled a number of surveys, around a fifth of men over the age of 50 complain about a loss of potency, sex drive, and morning erections, along with mild to moderate depression, irritability, and an earlier-than-usual decline in memory, and concentration. And yet the idea that this forms some kind of syndrome comparable to the menopause – otherwise known as the andropause – is too frequently dismissed out of hand by most doctors.

THE THYROID HORMONE, THYROXINE

There has been increasing interest in thyroid function in the elderly because of association of thyroid status with disability, cognitive function, cardiovascular disease risk, and longevity.

The effects of overt thyroid dysfunction are well documented in all age groups. The effects of subclinical thyroid disease in elderly population are still unclear, mainly due to lack of Randomised Control Trials (RCTs). In this paper, we evaluate the evidence about association of subclinical thyroid disease in the elderly with adverse outcomes and the evidence regarding intervention in this particular age group.

Thyroxine is the main hormone secreted into the bloodstream by the thyroid gland. It is the inactive form and most of it is converted to an active form called triiodothyronine by organs such as the liver and kidneys. Thyroid hormones play vital roles in regulating the body's metabolic rate, heart and digestive functions, muscle control, brain development and maintenance of bones.

The production and release of thyroid hormones, thyroxine and triiodothyronine, is controlled by a feedback loop system which involves the hypothalamus in the brain and the pituitary and thyroid glands. The hypothalamus secretes thyrotropin-releasing hormone which, in turn, stimulates the pituitary gland to produce thyroid stimulating hormone. This hormone stimulates the production of the thyroid hormones, thyroxine and triiodothyronine, by the thyroid gland.

This hormone production system is regulated by a negative feedback loop so that when the levels of the thyroid hormones, thyroxine and triiodothyronine increase, they prevent the release of both thyrotropin-releasing hormone and thyroid stimulating hormone. This system allows the body to maintain a constant level of thyroid hormones in the body.

The release of too much thyroxine in the bloodstream is known as thyrotoxicosis. This may be caused by over activity of the thyroid gland (hyperthyroidism), as in Graves' disease, inflammation of the thyroid or a benign tumour. Thyrotoxicosis can be recognised by a goitre which is a swelling of the neck due to enlargement of the thyroid gland.

Other symptoms of thyrotoxicosis include:

- Intolerance to heat
- Weight loss
- Increased appetite
- Increased bowel movements
- Irregular menstrual cycle
- Rapid or irregular heartbeat
- Palpitations
- Tiredness
- Irritability
- Tremor
- Hair loss
- Retraction of the eyelids resulting in a 'staring' appearance

Too little production of thyroxine by the thyroid gland is known as hypothyroidism. It may be caused by autoimmune diseases, poor iodine intake or brought on by the use of certain drugs. Sometimes, the cause is unknown. Thyroid hormones are essential for physical and mental development so hypothyroidism during development or before birth and during childhood causes mental impairment and reduced physical growth.

Hypothyroidism in adults causes a decreased metabolic rate. This results in symptoms which include:

- Fatigue
- Intolerance of cold temperatures
- Low heart rate
- Weight gain

- Reduced appetite
- Poor memory
- Depression
- Stiffness of the muscles
- Infertility

Hormones affect almost every part of your system so, not surprisingly, when your levels drop too low you can suffer a confusingly wide range of symptoms – and most of these could also be caused by something else!

If you've been suffering from any of the following for a while, it's worth having your hormones checked to see if they could be contributing to:

- Anxiety, depression, irritability, and mood swings
- Increased pain, inflammation, and aching joints
- Insomnia, night sweats, and weight gain
- Thinner, older skin with more wrinkles
- Decreased libido and lack of energy, and drive
- Confusion and memory problems

Depending on your symptoms and test results, you may find real benefit in correcting the hormones that you are deficient in by using bio-identical hormones given in the dose equivalent to that which your body would normally make. I recommend that you are reassessed after three and six months, because some hormone imbalances will be corrected so that you won't need to keep taking as much. Will natural hormones extend your healthy lifespan? The odds are good, but there's no definitive proof yet.

No one wants to age but it is inevitable and seeing that there is no 'fountain of youth', the next best thing is healthy ageing… growing older but staying healthy.

As an anti-ageing doctor that is my main motivation for my patients.

SO HOW CAN WE AGE HEALTHILY?

Balancing and keeping your hormones balanced naturally is the key to healthy ageing.

Ageing doesn't happen just because our bodies get old. It happens because our brains stop producing a very important anti-ageing hormone - human growth hormone.

Human growth hormones (HGH) are produced naturally by the pituitary gland in your brain throughout your childhood and young adult years. The hormones work to help your body grow when you're young. They also strengthen your bones, maintain your skin tissues, and increase your muscle mass. When you reach your middle age years and beyond, this important anti-ageing hormone is produced less and less, and so you age. Your skin becomes weaker, your bones brittle, and you lose muscle mass.

It makes sense to think that if we found a way to maintain the output of this anti-ageing hormone produced by your brain, we could actually reverse the ageing process. That's why some people have dubbed HGH as the 'fountain of youth'.

These anti-ageing hormones have many benefits for your body, other than reversing the ageing process. They can help with strengthening the ligaments and other connective tissues in your body, and make you healthier by making your immune system stronger. When you have high levels of anti-ageing hormones in your body, your risk for certain diseases, including adult onset diabetes, becomes significantly lower.

How do we encourage anti-ageing hormones to be produced by our brains even when we reach middle age?

Do we inject ourselves with synthetic growth hormones?

How do we encourage natural anti-ageing hormones?

NATURAL GROWTH HORMONE BOOSTERS

Human growth hormone (HGH) plays a vital role in staying young. With age, the body naturally starts to produce less. The good news is that there are safe, natural methods to boost the release of HGH so you can retain your youthfulness.

NATURAL HGH BOOSTER #1: FENUGREEK

Early studies show that this vegetable, popular in Asia, stimulates the release of growth hormone and can boost energy levels. Steam fenugreek herbs or enjoy as a tea.

NATURAL HGH BOOSTER #2: L-ARGININE

This amino acid stimulates the release of the growth hormone from the pituitary gland. Take it in supplement form: 2 grams, three times a day.

NATURAL HGH BOOSTER #3: A SLEEP MASK

You release the most HGH while you sleep. Use a sleep mask to block out light, allowing melatonin, the sleep hormone, to surge, and get a deeper, more restorative sleep.

So, as you can see HGH is a vital component of the human endocrine system.

In adulthood, its presence leads to a healthier body composition and is responsible for such important jobs such as:

- Keeping your body lean
- Decreasing fat accumulation
- Strengthening your bones
- Protecting your organs from the decline that occurs with age
- Promoting more rapid hair and nail growth
- Improving circulation
- Giving a more favourable cholesterol profile
- Helping protect you from the consequences of aging

Unfortunately, natural production of HGH declines as you get older. This progressive deficiency, beginning, for most, in our 20s, leads to a reduction in lean body mass and bone mineral density, an increase in body fat – especially abdominal, and a worsened cardiovascular risk profile.

All in all, you begin to look and feel older as HGH declines.

I treat Adult Growth Hormone Deficiency (AGHD) as well as other hormonal deficiencies in my practice. The easiest and most accurate way to test for HGH deficiency is with a blood test called an IGF-1. IGF-1 is a hormone produced in response to HGH secretion by the pituitary gland. It is the best marker of the status of secretion of HGH, and a low value less than 200 is indicative of growth hormone deficiency. Levels below 200 are generally considered to be in the deficient state.

The quickest and most effective way to increase HGH levels is with a daily injection of HGH. Numerous studies have shown that replacement therapy is beneficial and such treatment has become recognised as standard practice. In adults, HGH replacement therapy will often be maintained for many years.

Exercise, stress, emotional excitement, diet and ageing all affect the quantity of HGH production.

Certain lifestyle factors, such as sleep and stress management, our specific nutritional plan and our scientifically-based exercise plan, cause the pituitary to secrete more HGH.

Here are 10 of the most effective ways to increase HGH production naturally:

HIGH INTENSITY BURST TRAINING
The type of training in which one's heart rate bursts above their anaerobic threshold (best established by VO2 max testing) for 30 second

intervals five or more times in a workout. This engages super-fast twitch muscle fibres, which release HGH naturally.

GET ADEQUATE SLEEP
Getting 8 hours per night optimises production of HGH.

MELATONIN
Take 0.5 to 5 mg of melatonin before bed. Melatonin has been shown to increase growth hormone levels by up to 157%.

GABA
Take 1.5 to 3 g of GABA immediately before bed. GABA, or gamma aminobutyric acid, has been shown to increase growth hormone production by 200%.

EAT HIGH QUALITY PROTEIN
Consume a high-protein, low-carbohydrate snack before going to bed. The amino acids will help to boost HGH, while avoiding too many carbohydrates will keep insulin levels low so that it cannot inhibit growth hormone from doing its work.

VITAMIN D
Optimise Vitamin D levels at 50 - 75ng/mL.

AVOID SUGAR AFTER WORKOUTS
Consuming sugar (especially fructose) within two hours post-workout will cause your hypothalamus to release somatostatin, which will

decrease your production of HGH. Simple sugars that are high-gly-caemic also spike insulin levels. Not only does this lead to body fat storage, but it severely decreases the release of growth hormone.

L-ARGININE AND L-LYSINE

The combination of these two amino acids together before exercise and sleep has been shown to increase growth hormone production by up to 700%. Take 3 to 5g for optimal results.

GLUTAMINE

Take 2 to 10g of glutamine after a workout or before bed. Glutamine may boost HGH levels, according to a study conducted by research-ers at the Louisiana State College of Medicine. They discovered that subjects consuming 2g of glutamine experienced increases in HGH levels. Their findings were reported in the 1995 issue of The American Journal of Clinical Nutrition.

ALPHA-GLYCERYLPHOSPHORYLCHOLINE (A-GPC)

A-GPC might increase HGH levels, according to a study published in the September 2008 issue of the Journal of the International Society of Sports Nutrition. Researchers at the Center for Applied Health Science Research observed that subjects taking 600mg of A-GPC two hours before resistance exercise had higher HGH levels post-exercise compared with those who consumed a placebo.

CHAPTER 4

Your hormone-friendly diet

AND SUPPORTING SUPPLEMENTS

GL stands for Glycaemic Load. It's a unit of measurement that tells you exactly what a particular food will do to your blood sugar. Foods with a high GL have a greater effect on your blood sugar, which isn't desirable. Foods with a low GL encourage the body to burn fat, which is what we're aiming for.

Keeping your blood sugar balanced is the concept at the heart of the low GL diet – sustainable weight loss will follow.

When your blood sugar level increases, the hormone insulin is released into the bloodstream to remove the glucose (sugar). Some glucose goes to the brain and muscles where it's used as an energy fuel, but any excess goes to the liver where it's turned into fat and stored, causing you to gain weight. Insulin is known as the fat-storing hormone.

The glycaemic load (GL) is based on the glycaemic index (GI). Put simply, the glycaemic index of a food tells you whether the carbohydrate in a food is fast or slow releasing (fast is bad, slow is good). What it doesn't tell you, is exactly how much of the food is carbohydrate.

Glycaemic load on the other hand tells you both the type and amount of carbohydrate in the food and what that particular carbohydrate does to your blood sugar.

3 GOLDEN RULES

For balancing your blood sugar, there are only three rules:
- Eat 45GLs daily to lose weight or 65GLs to maintain weight
- Eat carbohydrate with protein
- Eat little and often

5 SIMPLE PRINCIPLES

- Balance your blood sugar
- Eat good fats, avoid bad fats
- Eliminate allergies
- Supplement for success
- Exercise for at least 15 minutes daily

THE PROTEIN-CARBOHYDRATE CONNECTION

There are two ways to achieve a low GL meal. The first is to avoid carbohydrates altogether and eat lots of protein and fat (Atkins style – not recommended, in my opinion).

The other is to have some carbohydrates, but only those that release their sugar content slowly (low GL) and to always eat them with protein (my preferred option).

The glycemic index range is as follows:
- Low GI = 55 or less
- Medium GI = 56 - 69
- High GI = 70 or more

BREAKFAST CEREAL

Low GI			Medium GI			High GI		
All-bran	–	30	Bran Buds	–	58	Cornflakes	–	80
All-bran (US)	–	50	Mini Wheats	–	58	Sultana Bran	–	73
Oat bran	–	50	Nutrigrain	–	66	Branflakes	–	74
Rolled Oats	–	51	Shredded Wheat	–	67	Coco Pops	–	77
Special K	–	54	Porridge Oats	–	63	Puffed Wheat	–	80
Natural Muesli	–	40	Special K (US)	–	69	Oats - honey bake	–	77
Porridge	–	58				Team	–	82
						Total	–	76
						Cheerios	–	74
						Rice Krispies	–	82
						Weetbix	–	74

BREAD

Low GI			Medium GI			High GI		
Soya and Linseed	–	36	Croissant	–	67	White	–	80
Wholegrain			Hamburger			Bagel	–	73
Pumpernickel	–	46	bun	–	61	French Baguette	–	74
Heavy Mixed Grain	–	45	Pita, white	–	57			
Whole Wheat	–	49	Wholemeal					
Sourdough Rye	–	48	Rye	–	62			
Sourdough Wheat	–	54						

VEGETABLES

Low GI			Medium GI			High GI		
Frozen Green Peas	–	39	Beetroot	–	64	Pumpkin	–	75
Frozen Sweet Corn	–	47				Parsnips	–	97
Raw Carrots	–	16						
Boiled Carrots	–	41						
Eggplant/Aubergine	–	15						
Broccoli	–	10						
Cauliflower	–	15						
Cabbage	–	10						
Mushrooms	–	10						
Tomatoes	–	15						
Chillies	–	10						
Lettuce	–	10						
Green Beans	–	15						
Red Peppers	–	10						
Onions	–	10						

STAPLES

Low GI		Medium GI		High GI	
Wheat Pasta	54	Basmati Rice	– 58	Instant White Rice	– 87
Shapes	– 54	Couscous	– 61	Glutinous Rice	– 86
New Potatoes	– 39	Cornmeal	– 68	Short Grain White	
Meat Ravioli	– 32	Taco Shells	– 68	Rice	– 83
Spaghetti	– 50	Gnocchi	– 68	Tapioca	– 70
Tortellini (Cheese)	– 32	Canned		Fresh Mashed	
Egg Fettuccini	– 50	Potatoes	– 61	Potatoes	– 73
Brown Rice	– 51	Chinese (Rice)		French Fries	– 75
Buckwheat	– 50	Vermicelli	– 58	Instant Mashed	
White long	22	Baked Potatoes	– 60	Potatoes	– 80
grain rice	– 35	Wild Rice	– 57		
Pearled Barley	– 48				
Yam	– 47				
Sweet Potatoes	– 30				
Instant Noodles	–				
Wheat tortilla	–				

FOODS

Low GI		Medium GI		High GI	
Slim-Fast meal replacement	– 27	Ryvita	– 63	Pretzels	– 83
Snickers Bar (high fat)	– 41	Digestives	– 59	Water Crackers	– 78
Nut & Seed Muesli Bar	– 49	Blueberry	59	Rice cakes	– 87
Sponge Cake	– 46	muffin	– 58	Puffed	81
Nutella	– 33	Honey	–	Crispbread	– 76
Milk Chocolate	– 42			Donuts	– 92
Hummus	– 6			Scones	– 68
Peanuts	– 13			Maple flavoured	
Walnuts	– 15			syrup	–
Cashew Nuts	– 25				
Nuts and Raisins	– 21				
Jam	– 51				
Corn Chips	– 42				
Oatmeal Crackers	– 55				

LEGUMES (BEANS)

Low GI		Medium GI	
Kidney Beans (canned)	– 52	Beans in Tomato Sauce	– 56
Butter Beans	– 36		
Chick Peas	– 42		
Haricot/Navy Beans	– 31		
Lentils, Red	– 21		
Lentils, Green	– 30		
Pinto Beans	– 45		
Blackeyed Beans	– 50		
Yellow Split Peas	– 32		

FRUIT

Low GI			Medium GI			High GI		
Cherries	–	22	Mango	–	60	Watermelon	–	80
Plums	–	24	Sultanas	–	56	Dates	–	103
Grapefruit	–	25	Bananas	–	58			
Peaches	–	28	Raisins	–	64			
Peach, canned in		30	Papaya	–	60			
natural juice	–	34	Figs	–	61			
Apples	–	41	Pineapple	–	66			
Pears	–	32						
Dried Apricots	–	43						
Grapes	–	45						
Coconut	–	41						
Coconut Milk	–	47						
Kiwi Fruit	–	40						
Oranges	–	40						
Strawberries	–	29						
Prunes	–							

DAIRY

Low GI			Medium GI		
Whole milk	–	31	Ice cream	–	62
Skimmed milk	–	32			
Chocolate milk	–	42			
Sweetened yoghurt	–	33			
Artificially Sweetened Yoghurt	–	23			
Custard	–	35			
Soy Milk	–	44			

Protein helps to slow down the release of sugar from carbohydrates and has virtually no effect on blood sugar.

What about fat?

While fats don't have any effect on blood sugar, the amount and type of fat you eat will still affect how much weight you lose. Saturated fat is easily stored in the body as fat, so should be avoided. Essential fats (omega 3 and 6) are crucial to your health and need to feature in your diet daily.

You will find omega 3 fatty acids in oily fish such as salmon, trout, mackerel, and sardines, as well as in flax and pumpkin seeds. Omega 6 fatty acids are found in nuts and seeds as well as in evening primrose oil, corn oil, and soya oil.

THE IMPORTANCE OF EXERCISE

Exercise is the fastest way to improve your metabolic rate. Muscle burns more energy than fat, so the less muscle you have the slower your metabolism. Combining low GL eating with regular exercise is important for a successful diet.

LOW GL BENEFITS

- **You won't feel hungry** – while a restricted diet will not fully satisfy your appetite, from day one the low GL diet recommends foods designed to satisfy your appetite and leave you feeling full.

- **It is safe** – unlike highly restrictive diets, the only side effect of a low GL diet is added health.

- **It's enjoyable and delicious** – no food groups are excluded on the low GL diet so you don't have to fight to stay on track.

You'll feel great – a low GL diet works with your body, not against it.

If you don't eat foods with the nutrients you need, your body cannot produce hormones correctly or maintain hormonal balance because it doesn't have the building blocks to do so.

Whatever you're eating is either helping hormonal production, or causing unpredictable imbalances.

The human body needs a balance of all three macronutrients, carbohydrates, protein, and especially fat.

Fat is one of the most crucial elements for hormonal balance. For years, we've been told that fat-free is good, while cholesterol and saturated fat are bad. This is a dangerous lie. Healthy fat is the raw material that we need to produce and maintain proper hormone function.

Here's why: hormones are produced using certain fatty acids and cholesterol, so if we're missing these nutrients, hormone problems arise simply because the body doesn't have the nutrients it needs to make them. Our body needs certain fats for rebuilding cells and stabilising hormones. This is especially important for the female reproductive system.

HOW TO EAT FOR HORMONAL BALANCE

Basing meals off clean protein, hormone-balancing healthy fats, anti-oxidant-rich vegetables and healing herbs will help your body thrive.

Choose one food from each category for an easy, hormone-balancing, skin-healing, meal.

1. CLEAN PROTEIN

- Soaked or sprouted nuts
- Beans
- Seeds
- Quinoa
- Lentils
- Organic pasture-raised/grass-fed chicken, turkey, beef, venison, and eggs
- Wild caught fish

2. HORMONE-BALANCING HEALTHY FATS

Coconut oil (and all coconut products for that matter) contains lauric acid, which is incredibly healing to the skin and extremely beneficial for hormonal production. It also kills bad bacteria and viruses in the body, provides a quick source of energy, is easy to digest, and speeds up metabolism.

Avocados are rich in healthy fat that helps our body absorb and use nutrients. They are also full of fibre, potassium, magnesium vitamin E, B-vitamins, and folic acid - all essential for maintaining hormonal balance in the body.

Raw butter provides a rich source of fat-soluble vitamins A, D, E and K2. These nutrients are key building blocks for hormonal production.

Butter provides great amounts of short- and medium-chain fatty acids, which support immune function, boost metabolism and have antimicrobial properties; meaning, they fight against bad bacteria and viruses in the body.

Egg yolks are rich in countless vitamins and minerals including: A, D, E, B2, B6, B9, iron, calcium, phosphorous, potassium and choline which all contribute to a healthy reproductive system, hormonal balance, and healthy skin. The choline and iodine in egg yolks are also crucial for making healthy thyroid hormones.

Nuts and seeds. Soaked nuts and seeds, olives and olive oil, fermented cod liver oil, hempseed oil, and flaxseed oil.

3. ANTIOXIDANT-RICH VEGETABLES

Look for anything dark green: asparagus, broccoli, spinach, collard greens, cabbage, cucumbers, kale and cilantro.

Opt for brightly coloured veggies: green, red, yellow, and orange bell peppers, red cabbage, red/white onions, tomatoes, and carrots.

Don't overlook starchy vegetables: sweet potatoes, pumpkin, beetroot, artichokes, butternut, squash, and turnips.

4. HEALING SPICES & HERBS

- Cinnamon
- Turmeric
- Cayenne
- Cumin

- Garlic
- Ginger

If your body has the nutrients it needs to be in hormonal balance, it will be. You'll experience glowing skin, stable moods, fertility, and consistent energy.

Your body has an incredible ability to heal and be in balance, when given the nutrients it needs to flourish.

WHAT TO AVOID IN YOUR DIET

Artificial sweeteners and MSG: Artificial sweeteners are the Joker of the food industry and aren't as sweet as you might think. Sucralose, better known as Canderel, is created by chlorinating sucrose replacing hydroxyl with chlorine, which is a known carcinogen. As well as being a health risk, sucralose appears to actually cause weight gain, possibly because it still triggers the release of insulin, which is thought to induce people to actually eat more.

In a report from an official United States Air Force publication, pilots were warned not to consume aspartame. The report stated, 'Aspartame has been investigated as a possible cause of brain tumours, mental retardation, birth defects, epilepsy, Parkinson's Disease, fibromyalgia, and diabetes.'

To date the FDA has made no move to regulate aspartame, which is sold as NutraSweet or

Equal. Monosodium glutamate (MSG) is used as a flavour-enhancer, yet it can cause side effects such as sweating, nausea, headaches, and even numbness in the face and neck. It has also been linked to weight gain, according to studies by the University of North Carolina who found that those who consumed MSG on a regular basis were more likely to be overweight or obese.

Processed grains and sugar: Processed grains and sugars are like Kryptonite to the human body. White bread, pasta, rice, sugary cereals, pastries, crackers, and sweets aren't only non-nutritious, they are actually anti-nutrients. These foods that are sugar based or immediately turn into sugar once ingested into your system, system actually leach vitamins out of your cells.

Ever hit the 2 p.m. 'carb coma' at your workplace from eating a big carbohydrate loaded lunch?

That is in part because processed grains and sugars are actually sucking the life out of you!

Your body is designed to be a hunter-gatherer, yet in modern-day diets they are just high in carbohydrates, processed grains, and sugar. Where you consume far too much bread, cereal, pasta, rice, and cakes than you should - your body is protesting!

Those who suffer from being overweight, fatigue, insomnia, depression, foggy brain, bloating, low blood sugar, high blood pressure or high triglycerides need to change their diet quickly before it literally becomes the death of you.

Refined carbohydrates are derived from processed grains which have had most of the nutrients removed. Refined grains are the main ingredients in bread, cereal, and pasta.

They're known as 'empty calories' as they're stripped of nutrients, fibre, and vitamins.

B-COMPLEX VITAMINS
Folic acid, vitamin B6 and vitamin B12

Cardiovascular disease, the number-one killer of men and women claims the lives of almost 40% of people who die each year in South Africa. With 6.3 million people living with high blood pressure, South Africa has one of the highest cardiovascular disease rates in the world; about half of all deaths are due to heart disease and stroke. Statistics show that about 130 heart attacks and 240 strokes occur daily in South Africa.

Homocysteine a non-essential, sulphur-containing amino acid is an independent marker of risk for the development of cardiovascular disease.

I recommend that you reduce homocysteine levels by taking folic acid, vitamin B6 and vitamin B12. Some researchers consider homocysteine as important a cardiovascular risk factor as low-density lipoprotein (LDL or the 'bad' cholesterol). Homocysteine can make blood clot more easily than normal, increasing the risk of both heart attack and death by heart attack. Inadequate levels of folic acid, and vitamins B6 and B12 can lead to increased homocysteine levels.

ANTI-AGEING SUPPLEMENTS

COENZYME Q10

Coenzyme Q10 (CoQ10) is an essential component of healthy mitochondrial function. It is incorporated into cells' mitochondria throughout the body where it facilitates and regulates the oxidation of fats and sugars into energy. Ageing humans have been found to have over 50% less CoQ10 on average compared to that of young adults. This finding makes CoQ10 one of the most important nutrients for people over 30 to supplement with. About 95% of cellular energy is produced in the mitochondria. The mitochondria are the cells 'energy powerhouses' and many maladies have been referred to as 'mitochondrial disorders'. A growing body of scientific research links a deficiency of CoQ10 to age-related mitochondrial disorders.

ACETYL-L-CARNITINE ARGINATE

The amino acid acetyl-L-carnitine boosts mitochondrial energy production through its ability to facilitate fatty acid transport and oxidation in the cell. My patients have been supplementing with acetyl-L-carnitine for years and deriving the many benefits this form of carnitine has shown in published studies. With the discovery of acetyl-L-carnitine arginate the benefits of acetyl-L-carnitine can now be greatly augmented. Acetyl-L-carnitine arginate is a patented form of carnitine that stimulates the growth of neurites in the brain. Studies show that acetyl-L-carnitine-arginate stimulates the growth of new neurites by an astounding 19.5%. Acetyl-L-carnitine-arginate acts together with acetyl-L-carnitine to increase neurite outgrowth.

CARNOSINE

Carnosine is a multifunctional dipeptide made up of a chemical combination of the amino acids beta-alanine and L-histidine. It is found both in food and in the human body. Long-lived cells such as nerve cells (neurons) and muscle cells (myocytes) contain high levels of carnosine.

Muscular levels of carnosine correlate with the maximum life spans of animals. Carnosine levels decline with age. Muscle levels decline 63% from age 10 to age 70, which may account for the normal age-related decline in muscle mass and function. Since carnosine acts as a pH buffer, it can keep on protecting muscle cell membranes from oxidation under the acidic conditions of muscular exertion.

Carnosine enables the heart muscle to contract more efficiently through enhancement of calcium response in heart myocytes. Ageing causes irreversible damage to the body's proteins. The underlying mechanism behind this damage is glycation. A simple definition of glycation is the cross-linking of proteins and sugars to form non-functioning structures in the body. The process of glycation can be superficially seen as unsightly wrinkled skin. Glycation is also an underlying cause of age-related catastrophes including neurological, vascular and eye disorders.

Carnosine is a unique dipeptide that interferes with the glycation process.

FISH OIL

Studies on omega-3 fatty acids are so impressive that an agency of the National Institutes of Health published a report stating that fish oil can help reduce deaths from heart disease.

The FDA itself states supportive but not conclusive research shows that consumption of EPA and DHA omega-3 fatty acids may actually reduce the risk of coronary heart disease. There are several mechanisms attributed to fish oil's beneficial effects. The latest government report cites the triglyceride-lowering effects of fish oil on reducing heart and blood vessel disorders.

Another beneficial mechanism of fish oil is to protect healthy blood flow in arteries.

GREEN TEA EXTRACT

What makes green tea extract such an important nutrient are the large volumes of published scientific findings that validate its multiple biological benefits. The most significant findings involve studies showing that green tea extract helps maintain cellular DNA and membrane structural integrity. Decades of research shows that green tea inhibits the development of undesirable cell colonies. The active constituents in green tea are powerful antioxidants called polyphenols (catechins) and flavonols. Several catechins are present in green tea and account for the bulk of favourable research reports. Epigallocatechin gallate (EGCG) is the most powerful of these catechins. EGCG functions as an antioxidant that is about 25-100 times more potent than vitamins C and E.

One cup of green tea may provide 10-40mg of polyphenols and has antioxidant effects that are greater than a serving of broccoli, spinach, carrots, or strawberries. Theoretically, the high antioxidant activity of green tea makes it beneficial for protecting the body from oxidative damage due to free radicals.

LIPOIC ACID

Lipoic acid is a highly potent antioxidant that counteracts reactive free radicals in the mitochondria, the power plants of cells, where energy for all cellular activities is generated.

Some scientists believe that mitochondrial free radicals play an important role in human ageing, and have theorised that extra amounts of free-radical inhibiting compounds such as lipoic acid may be able to help slow ageing.

Lipoic acid is also effective in recycling other antioxidants such as vitamin E back into their original form after they detoxify free radicals. There is also evidence that lipoic acid can reduce glycation damage due to excess glucose in the blood, which may be involved in ageing.

Lipoic acid consists of two different forms (isomers) that have vastly different properties. The 'R' form is the biologically active component (native to the body) that is responsible for lipoic acid's phenomenal antioxidant effect.

L-ALPHA-GLYCERYLPHOSPHORYLCHOLINE (GPC)

L-alpha glycerylphosphoryl-choline (GPC) is a product of phosphatidylcholine and helps to boost acetylcholine. It aids in the synthesis of several brain phospholipids, which increases the availability of acetylcholine in various brain tissues. The GPC form of choline has been shown in studies to help protect against cognitive decline normally seen in ageing.

PYRROLOQUINOLINE QUINONE (PQQ)

Until recently, the only options for ageing individuals to promote replenishment of the declining numbers of mitochondria in their bodies were long-term calorie restriction or exhaustive physical activity—difficult or impractical for most aging people. Now there is a viable alternative. PQQ activates genes that promote the formation of new mitochondria. It also beneficially interacts with genes directly involved in mitochondrial health. These same genes support healthy body weight, normal fat and sugar metabolism, and youthful cellular proliferation.

RESVERATROL

Findings from published scientific literature indicate that resveratrol may be the most effective compound for maintaining optimal health and promoting longevity. Resveratrol is a phytoalexin, a polyphenolic compound which is produced by Vitis vinifera (common grape vine) as a response to attack by moulds.

Research showed that a combination of low-dose (20 mg) resveratrol plus Grape Seed extract mimicked many of the favourable gene expression changes seen in calorie-restricted animals. Other studies, however, indicate that higher doses may be needed to obtain all of resveratrol's positive benefits, including promoting healthy insulin sensitivity, enhanced mitochondrial function, reduced expression of inflammatory factors, and protection against the effects of a high-fat diet.

WHEY PROTEIN

Many people think of whey protein as a supplement only used by athletes wanting to increase their muscle mass. But evolving research suggests the branched-chain amino acids (BCAAs) leucine, isoleucine, and valine, and other fractions found in whey can mimic the longevity benefits of calorie restriction. Whey protein can also have a positive impact on muscle construction and immunity due to its BCAA profile and naturally occurring lactoferrin and immunoglobins.

CALORIE RESTRICTION

Since the 1930s it has been known that a diet restricted in calories, but otherwise rich in nutrients, dramatically extends the life span of experimental animals. Over two thousand studies have confirmed the effectiveness of calorie restriction, (or 'undernutrition without malnutrition', as Roy Walford calls it), in a wide variety of species.

While the effectiveness of this anti-ageing regimen is likely far greater than others currently available, the difficulty of the regimen for most people is also far greater. Serious life extensionists should nevertheless consider trying at least a mild version of the diet.

THE GUT

Hippocrates was once quoted as saying, 'All disease begins in the gut.' Time is proving Hippocrates to be a pretty smart guy. Science is even now linking poor gut health with a myriad of health problems.

From eczema to poor immune health, it seems that our gut health influences much more than we previously realised. If all disease begins in the gut, it is logical to realise that perhaps optimal health begins here as well.

You know that 'gut feeling'?

It is estimated that over three quarters of our immune system resides in our intestinal tract, with over 500 species of bacteria present.

Overall, there is ten times the number of bacteria in the body than actual human cells, and this colonisation of bacteria (good or bad) can weigh up to 1.5kg. With such a large concentration of bacteria in our bodies, it is logical that we depend rather heavily on them for health.

Traditional diets around the world have typically included raw and fermented foods teeming with bacteria, including many beneficial strains. From yogurt, to kefir, to sauerkraut and fermented fish - cultures around the world are not afraid of some bacteria.

In our modern society, we've effectively managed to pasteurise, irradiate, and process out any naturally occurring beneficial bacteria while at the same time feeding harmful bacteria with a feast of processed starches and sugars.

On top of that, we sanitise our children from the moment they are born, afraid to ever let them encounter bacteria, good or bad, which are necessary for immune development. Besides the fact that research has found that antibacterial soap is no more beneficial than regular soap and water, and might actually be harmful. Raising our kids with 'hand sanitiser' in hand may not even let their digestive systems develop properly.

It has now been found that babies are born with a completely sterile digestive system, since *in utero*, they don't need gut bacteria for the breakdown of food as all nourishment comes from the mother. During the rather messy birth process, the baby's digestive system begins to colonise bacteria based on the mother's existing bacteria (good or bad!).

The baby's bacteria further develop during breastfeeding thanks to certain strains of immune boosting beneficial bacteria found only in breast milk. Since the baby depends on the birth process and on breast milk for this balance of bacteria, it makes sense that babies born naturally and then breastfed have lower rates of eczema, allergies, and illness.

Babies born by caesarean, or who are formula fed, are not doomed from the start, but it is good for parents to be aware of this need for probiotic bacteria and consider supplementation and natural sources.

After the infant stage, toddlers naturally supplement probiotics by putting everything, dirt included, into their mouths. If given the proper resources, these beneficial bacteria grow and flourish, boosting immunity and allowing proper breakdown of food.

Unfortunately, this isn't the norm anymore. More often, the balance of good bacteria is altered by an abundance of starches, sugars, and vegetable oils in the diet, or destroyed completely by antibiotic use or other pharmaceuticals. Lack of exposure to bacteria in the environment and in food further aggravates this problem.

In fact, in our bleach-cleaned world of processed foods, many of us might benefit from a good dose of healthy bacteria. The digestive tract has almost as many nerve cells as the spinal cord, and research is increasingly linking digestive health to overall health.

Beneficial bacteria are necessary to properly digest food (especially starches) and to absorb nutrients. Bacteria play a big role in overall immunity. With the rise of digestive problems like IBS, Crohn's disease, coeliac disease, colitis and allergies, a good dose of beneficial bacteria certainly wouldn't hurt.

The good news is that while outside sources are constantly working against our good bacteria these days, there are ways to boost good bacteria naturally, even for those of us not nursing or fond of eating dirt.

An ounce of prevention...

One of the best ways to keep beneficial bacteria from becoming depleted is to avoid the things that deplete it in the first place, including:

- Antibiotic use (especially if it can be avoided or natural alternatives can be used)
- Use of antibacterial soap
- Overuse of harsh cleaning chemicals to sanitise
- Consumption of processed and refined foods
- Consumption of sugars or excess of starches
- Any sources of stress on the body that can be avoided (e.g. lack of sleep or overexertion)

Fortunately, even if you've depleted your beneficial bacteria by some of the methods above, there are ways to increase it and help balance the bacteria in your digestive system. Chances are, unless you already consume a lot of fermented foods, garden barefoot a lot and eat some dirt, your probiotic balance could use a boost.

Here are some tips for boosting your probiotic gut balance:

1. **Don't eat sugars, grains, excess starches or processed vegetable oils.** These foods deplete beneficial bacteria very quickly and can consequently suppress immunity and lead to a variety of health problems. There is no need to eat these foods, especially in processed form, so for the sake of your gut... avoid them!

2. **Eat lots of real foods.** Eating foods like vegetables, proteins, and fats will help support beneficial bacteria that feed on certain types of fibre in foods like veggies. They will also support the body in culturing additional good bacteria.

3. **Consume fermented foods and drinks.** Foods like sauerkraut, kimchi, fermented salsa, fermented veggies, natural yogurt, kefir, and naturally aged cheeses are natural sources of probiotics and eating a variety of these will help get in all the beneficial strains of bacteria. Cultured drinks like kombucha and water or milk kefir also provide probiotics.

4. **Use natural soap and water instead of antibacterial.** Antibacterial soap kills bacteria, good or bad, and some suggest that overuse of antibacterial soap may be contributing to the rise in resistant strains of bacteria like MRSA. Use a quality natural soap and warm water to clean hands.

5. **Start gardening.** Believe it or not, the benefits of dirt that rings true for kids are also beneficial for adults. If you aren't fond of mud pies, take up gardening. It is a way to get your vitamin D3 and probiotics in, whilst producing your own food… a win-win!

6. **Don't overuse antibiotics.** There are certainly cases when it is best to use antibiotics, but for mild illnesses that can be left to run their course or treated naturally, consider skipping the antibiotics, which will deplete all gut bacteria, including the beneficial strains. If you do need to take antibiotics, make sure to take a high quality probiotic at the same time and for awhile afterward, to help replenish bacteria.

7. **Take a probiotic supplement.** Many of us need more help in the probiotic department then simple dietary changes can provide. That being said, supplementing probiotics without a change in diet and lifestyle is just a waste of money! If you are already eating real foods including fermented foods/drinks and using other ways to replenish your bacteria, consider supplementing probiotics, at least for a while. This is also an important recommendation if you are currently using, or have recently used antibiotics. Children with eczema, allergies, digestive disturbances or those who were formula fed can often benefit from probiotics as well.

8. **Try the GAPS or SCD diet.** These diets are specifically focused on healing and rebuilding a digestive system that has been harmed over time, resulting in a leaky gut or an autoimmune disease. If

you have specific or acute symptoms, one of these diets may be the fastest/best way to help your body recover.

With so many things attacking our digestive system it would seem like an almost impossible task to try and restore its health. Luckily, with a bit of planning and time, it is possible to restore your gastrointestinal tract to optimal health. Healing the gut lining will allow your body to build a strong immune system again and produce the right amount of neurotransmitters so that you will feel well again.

ADOPTING A NEW APPROACH TO THE FOODS YOU CONSUME

This can be done by starting with the 'Four R's - remove, repair, restore, and replace.

STEP 1: REMOVE

In this first step we remove the offending foods and toxins from your diet that could be acting as stressors on your system. This means caffeine, alcohol, processed foods, bad fats, and any other foods you think may be causing issues, like gluten and dairy. All of these irritate the gut in some form and create an inflammatory response.

STEP 2: REPAIR

The next step is to begin to repair the gut and heal the damaged intestinal lining. You do this by consuming an unprocessed diet and giving your body time to rest by providing it with substances that are known to heal the gut, like L-glutamine, omega-3 fatty acids, zinc, antioxidants (in the form of vitamins A, C, and E), quercitin, aloe vera, and turmeric.

STEP 3: RESTORE

This involves the restoration of your gut's optimal bacterial flora population. This is done with the introduction of probiotics like Lactobacillus acidophilus and Bifidobacterium lactis.

A probiotic is a good bacteria and is ingested to help reinforce and maintain a healthy gastrointestinal tract and to help fight illness. In general a healthy lower intestinal tract should contain around 85% good bacteria. This helps to combat any overgrowth of bad bacteria.

Unfortunately, in most people these percentages are skewed and this allows for the gut health to drastically decline. The human gut is home to bad bacteria like salmonella and clostridium, which is fine as long as they are kept in order and don't get out of control.

STEP 4: REPLACE

This involves getting your bile salts, digestive enzymes, and hydrochloric acid levels to optimal levels to maintain and promote healthy digestion. This can be done by supplementing with digestive enzymes and organic salt to help make sure you have enough hydrochloric acid.

Recommended Foods and Supplements

L-Glutamine helps to heal and seal the gut along with aiding in recovery after workouts, so it's a double whammy supplement.

Quality Fish Oil preferably a liquid, not capsule, if you can stand the taste. This helps reduce inflammation, balance hormones, and supports the immune system.

Probiotics provide live strains of good bacteria to help bolster your defences.

Cinnamon can help to improve digestion and, as an added bonus, is great at balancing blood sugar levels.

Mint is great at soothing the stomach and can help to relax the gastrointestinal tract.

Zinc is very important as it is utilised to form digestive enzymes and also used in regulating hormones.

Prebiotics in the form of fermented foods help to feed friendly bacteria and allow them to thrive in a healthy environment. Fermented foods include bio-available yogurt, kefir, kimchi, and sauerkraut.

PH Balancing or Alkaline Foods - Anything green is generally okay, like kale, spinach, broccoli, wheatgrass, parsley, chlorella, and spirulina. These are all great at keeping high stomach acid levels in order.

So, remember with a bit of time and work on your part you can obtain optimal gut health, which will make sure that all that hard earned work in and out of the gym pays off and isn't wasted down the toilet.

A SIMPLE GUT HEALTH DIET

Foods to include and exclude during your 21-day programme

The set dietary list is designed to avoid the major foods that cause digestive problems and gut dysfunction.

Some foods, like beans and certain fruits, have been excluded from the diet because they are difficult to digest or are high in sugar, even though they are often a staple of a healthy diet.

Eat

- Greens and fresh vegetables
- Fresh and frozen berries
- Wild fish
- Grass-fed meats
- Organic or pasture-raised eggs
- Lentils, quinoa*
- Fermented foods (kimchi, sauerkraut)
- Nuts, seeds and nut butters**
- Coconut oil, olive oil
- Avocado

*Go easy on these, only a side serving a day.

**Go easy on nuts, only a handful a day.

Don't eat
- Gluten
- Dairy
- Processed sugar
- Alcohol
- Caffeine (coffee, soda, black tea)
- Beans, rice
- Soy, corn
- Potatoes
- Almost all fruits

THE MEAL PLAN

BREAKFAST

Gut Shake: 1 Protein powder with your choice of ingredients. Examples are almond or coconut milk, additional protein sources like nut butters (which also contain good fibre), a handful of greens like baby spinach and berries.

LUNCH

Prepare a hearty solid meal packed full of nutrients, healthy fats and protein including dark leafy greens (cooked or raw), healthy fats like avocado and coconut oil, and quality protein like fish, chicken, or turkey.

DINNER

Prepare a starter-sized salad with healthy fats and quality protein. This doesn't have to be a cold salad. Stir-fries and soups, that are largely vegetable-focused can work too, (but still make sure to include healthy fats and proteins).

After dinner take a ten minute walk, this helps aid digestion and bowel movements, reduces stress, and allows reflection on the day.

Leave a twelve-hour window between your evening salad and your morning shake.

Do your best not to eat anything 2 hours before bed.

How to balance your hormones naturally

I KNOW THAT AFTER ALL this information that you have read it can be very overwhelming. But knowledge is power and with it you will be able to bring balance to your hormones and health.

THESE BASIC STEPS ARE MY GUIDE TO HEALTHY AGEING

- **Eat real food** - the body can't make hormones when it doesn't have the proper building blocks. Consume enough high quality proteins, beneficial fats and nutrient dense vegetables to give your body what it needs.
- **Part with plastics** - many plastics contain endocrine disrupting chemicals like BPA. Stick with glass or stainless steel for cooking baking and food storage. Switch to a safe, reusable water bottle.
- **Sleep** - sleep is vitally important for hormone balance, maintain a proper weight and blood sugar regulation. Make sleep a top priority every night.

- **Supplement wisely** - once food, sleep and environment are taken care of, consider hormone helping supplements like I have mentioned previously but especially omega 3, vitamin D3, and magnesium.
- **Limit caffeine** - too much caffeine can wreak havoc on the endocrine system, especially if there are other hormone stressors involved like pregnancy, presence of toxins, overweight, and stress.
- **Exercise carefully** - if you have adrenal or thyroid struggles, working out too much might make things worse instead of better. Always start with light exercise like walking swimming or bike riding and work up as you see what your body can handle.
- **Gut health** - looking after your gut is last on my list but it is the most important after you have tackled the other six. But with a good diet and proper supplements it is the easiest.

This is a sample menu guide only; it does not take into account your specific calorie and health needs, any allergies or food intolerances. Please replace with your choice to meet your needs, as closely as possible, of seasonal and available substitutes.

SAMPLE MENU

MONDAY

BREAKFAST	½ cup oats with a handful of almonds and ½ cup of milk
Late morning snack	2 carrots with ¼ cup hummus
LUNCH	1 grilled fish fillet with mixed vegetables
Afternoon snack	2 brown rice crackers with cottage cheese
DINNER	Roast chicken with mixed vegetables and roast pumpkin

TUESDAY

BREAKFAST	1 poached egg on a slice of Low GI toast with mushrooms and tomatoes with basil
Late morning snack	5 sticks of celery and 5 walnuts
LUNCH	Roast chicken breast with mixed salad
Afternoon snack	1 carrot with humus
DINNER	Lean pork fillet grilled with mushroom couscous and vegetables or salad

WEDNESDAY

BREAKFAST	½ cup oats with a handful of almonds and ½ cup of milk
Late morning snack	1 pear & 4 brazil nuts
LUNCH	1 ½ cups of lentil and vegetable soup
Afternoon snack	1 orange with 5 almonds
DINNER	100g lean steak with stir-fried vegetables and ½ cup of wild rice

THURSDAY

BREAKFAST	1 slice of Low GI toast with 1 cup of mushrooms, 2 spears of asparagus and baked beans
Late morning snack	1 cup of strawberries with a cup of plain yoghurt
LUNCH	Sliced left over steak into a whole wheat wrap with mixed vegetables and salad
Afternoon snack	1 apple with 5 almonds
DINNER	Grilled fish with salad and roasted baby potatoes

FRIDAY

BREAKFAST	Smoothie: ½ cup of plain yoghurt, ½ cup of milk, ½ a banana, ½ cup of berries with a serving of good protein powder
Late morning snack	5 sticks of celery and 5 walnuts
LUNCH	Mixed beans and vegetable salad
Afternoon snack	1 pear with 4 brazil nuts
DINNER	Lean lamb and vegetable curry on ½ cup of basmati

SATURDAY

BREAKFAST	1 poached egg on a slice of Low GI toast with mushrooms and tomatoes with basil
Late morning snack	1 brown rice cake with 1 teaspoon of cottage cheese and ½ a pear
LUNCH	Ham, tomato, lettuce and avocado sandwich on Low GI bread
Afternoon snack	5 sticks of celery and 5 walnuts
DINNER	Homemade burgers with lean minced meat on a whole wheat bun with roasted sweet potato wedges

SUNDAY

BREAKFAST	2 slices of Low GI baked French toast with 1 teaspoon of 100% fruit jam
Late morning snack	½ tin of tuna in water with fresh cucumber and tomato
LUNCH	Sunday roast lunch with the family
Afternoon snack	Cappuccino with a nut whole wheat muffin
DINNER	Lean sausages with mashed cauliflower and salad

Contact details

For more information on putting your specialist team together and for your supplement needs contact:

DR CRAIGE GOLDING

SPECIALIST PHYSICIAN

Tel: 011 058 7600

Fax: 086 577 6353

Email: patients@craigegolding.co.za

Glossary

ASPARTIC ACID
Aspartic Acid, also known as aspartate, is an excitatory neurotransmitter in the brainstem and spinal cord. Aspartic acid is the excitatory counterpart to glycine, an inhibitory neurotransmitter. Low levels have been linked to feelings of fatigue and low mood, whereas high levels have been linked to seizures and anxiousness.

5 ALPHA REDUCTASE
An enzyme that converts testosterone, the male sex hormone, into the more potent dihydrotestosterone (DHT).

ADRENAL FATIGUE
A putative health disorder in which the adrenal glands are claimed to be exhausted and unable to produce adequate quantities of hormones, primarily cortisol. Also called hypoadrenia and adrenal insufficiency.

AGELESS
Not ageing or appearing to age.

AGEING
Multidimensional process of physical, psychological and social change in humans over time.

ALDOSTERONE
A hormone produced by the cortex of the adrenal gland, instrumental in the regulation of sodium and potassium reabsorption by the cells of the tubular portion of the kidney.

ALOPECIA AREATA
Hair loss occurring in only one section.

ALZHEIMER'S DISEASE
Also called SDAT (senile dementia Alzheimer's type)

This disease is characterised by a general loss of intellectual ability and impairment of memory, judgment and abstract thinking, as well as changes in personality. Other symptoms include loss of speech, disorientation and apathy. Alzheimer's disease is the most common cause of dementia, rarely occurring before the age of 50. The disease takes from a few months to four or five years to progress to complete loss of intellectual function.

AMPHETAMINES
Any group of drugs that stimulate the central nervous system, resulting in elevated blood pressure, heart rate and other metabolic functions

ANABOLIC STEROIDS
A class of steroid hormones related to the hormone testosterone. They increase protein synthesis within cells, which results in the build-up of cellular tissue (anabolism), especially in the muscles.

ANDROGEN
A steroid hormone, such as testosterone or androsterone, that promotes male characteristics.

ANDROPAUSE
The male counterpart of menopause, when the production of testosterone decreases and there are accompanying mental symptoms.

ANAEMIA
A condition marked by a deficiency of red blood cells or of haemoglobin in the blood, resulting in pallor and weakness

ANTI-AGEING MEDICINE
Medicine focused on preventing, slowing, or reversing the effects of ageing and helping people live longer, healthier, happier lives.

ANXIETY
Distress or uneasiness of mind caused by fear of danger or misfortune; a state of apprehension.

AROMATASE
An enzyme or complex of enzymes that promotes the conversion of an androgen (like testosterone) into oestrogens (like oestradiol).

BASELINE
A basic standard or level; guideline that can serve as a comparison or control.

BENIGN PROSTATIC HYPERPLASIA (BPH)
The increased size of the prostate in middle-aged and elderly men. Also referred to as nodular hyperplasia, benign prostatic hypertrophy or benign enlargement of the prostate (BPE).

BINDERS
An ingredient used to bind together two or more other materials (ingredients) in mixtures: a binder used in medication.

BIO-AVAILABLE
The degree to which or rate at which a hormone or other substance is absorbed or becomes available at the site of physiological activity.

BIO-IDENTICAL
Identical to the substance in the human body; bio-identical oestrogen.

BIO-IDENTICAL HORMONE REPLACEMENT THERAPY (BHRT)
Used to describe hormone supplementation for female menopause with oestradiol and progesterone, or male menopause with testosterone, but can also include dehydroepiandrosterone (DHEA), oestriol or oestrone. BHRT is part of a growing practice of restorative endocrinology of restoring several well-known human hormones to optimal levels and effects with the use of bio-identical hormones.

BIO-IDENTICAL HORMONES

Substances with the exact same molecular structure as those made in the human body, which produce the same physiological responses as the body's natural hormones.

BLOOD TEST

A Laboratory analysis performed on a blood sample that is usually extracted from a vein in the arm using a needle, or via a finger prick.

C-REACTIVE PROTEIN (CRP)

An inflammatory marker – a protein that the body releases in response to inflammation. Thus, elevated levels of CRP in the blood mean that there is inflammation somewhere in the body. CRP is not normally present in the blood of a healthy patient. CRP levels can increase by as much as 1 000 times with inflammation. Conditions that commonly lead to marked changes in CRP include infection, trauma, surgery, burns, inflammatory conditions, and advanced cancer. Moderate changes occur after strenuous exercise, heatstroke, and childbirth. Psychological stress and some psychiatric illnesses can cause small changes in CRP levels. CRP is the only inflammatory marker that has been found to be an indicator of heart health. Therefore, doctors often carry out a CRP test at the same time as cholesterol and other lipid tests to help predict a patient's risk of heart attack.

CELL

A usually microscopic structure containing nuclear and cytoplasmic material enclosed by a semi-permeable membrane; the basic structural unit of all organisms.

CELL MEMBRANE

The interface between the cellular machinery inside the cell and the fluid outside. A semi-permeable lipid bilayer found in all cells containing biological molecules, primarily proteins and lipids.

CENTRAL SLEEP APNOEA

A central nervous system disorder in which the brain signal for breathing is delayed. Often caused by injury or disease affecting the brain stem.

CIRCADIAN RHYTHM
An approximate daily periodicity, a roughly 24-hour cycle in the biochemical, physiological or behavioural processes of living beings. These rhythms allow organisms to anticipate and prepare for precise and regular environmental changes.

COMPLETE BLOOD COUNT
A test that gives information about the cells in a person's blood including the white blood cells (leukocytes), red blood cells (erythrocytes) and platelets.

COMPOUNDING
To produce or create by combining two or more ingredients or parts: pharmacists compounding prescriptions.

COMPOUNDING PHARMACY
A specialised pharmacy that hand makes individualised bio-identical hormone prescriptions and other medicines.

CONVERT
To cause a substance to undergo a chemical change. (conversion)

CORPUS LUTEUM
A yellow, progesterone-secreting mass of cells that forms from an ovarian follicle after the release of a mature egg.

CORTISOL
A steroid hormone produced by the adrenal gland which regulates carbohydrate metabolism, stress and maintains blood pressure. Also called hydrocortisone.

COVALENT BONDS
A form of chemical bonding that is characterised by the sharing of pairs of electrons between atoms, or between atoms and other covalent bonds.

CREATININE
Creatinine is a normalising parameter used to calculate neurotransmitter levels. Creatinine is produced at a constant rate through the kidneys. Therefore, by using creatinine as the constant factor, spot urinary measurements can be performed without having to factor in the patient's hydration state, possible renal disorders or diuretic substances that may have been used.

DEFICIENCY
The amount lacked; a shortage: an oestrogen deficiency or vitamin deficiency.

DEGENERATIVE
Of, relating to, involving, or tending to cause degeneration; to diminish in quality, esp. for a former state of coherence, balance, integrity, etc.

DEHYDROEPIANDROSTERONE (DHEA)
A steroid hormone naturally produced by the adrenal glands and sold in synthetic form as a nutritional supplement.

DEPRESSION
A condition of general emotional dejection and withdrawal; sadness greater and more prolonged than that warranted by any objective reason.

DHT (DIHYDROTESTOSTERONE)
A conversion of testosterone that is considered to be an ageing-bio-marker. Among its affects are the appearance of body-hair, the loss of scalp hair and the onset of prostate gland problems.

DIAGNOSTIC TEST
Any kind of medical test performed to aid in the diagnosis or detection of disease or poor health.

DISORDER
A disturbance in physical or mental health, or functions.

DOMINO EFFECT
The cumulative effect that results when one event precipitates a series of like events.

DOPAMINE
Dopamine is an excitatory and inhibitory neurotransmitter, depending on the dopaminergic receptor it binds to. It is derived from the amino acid tyrosine. Dopamine is the precursor to norepinephrine and epinephrine, which are all catecholamines. The function of dopamine is diverse but plays a large role in the pleasure/reward pathway (addiction and thrills), memory, and motor control. Dopamine, like norepinephrine and epinephrine, is stored in vesicles in the axon terminal. Dopamine plays a significant role in the cardiovascular, renal, hormonal, and central nervous systems. The dopaminergic neurons have dendrites that extend into various regions of the brain, controlling different functions through the stimulation of adrenergic and dopaminergic receptors. Common symptoms with low dopamine levels are loss of motor control, addictions, cravings, compulsions, and loss of satisfaction. When dopamine levels are elevated symptoms may manifest in the form of anxiety or hyperactivity. Some therapies utilize L-DOPA for Parkinsonian symptoms which can also cause elevations in dopamine.

DOPAMINE METABOLITE
After neuronal dopamine is released it is inactivated primarily via reuptake mechanisms that remove it from the synapse and the extraneuronal space and return it to the presynaptic dopaminergic neuron or adjacent noradrenergic neurons.

Some of the enzymes that degrade dopamine are only found in specific regions of the body. As such some dopamine metabolites are only produced in specific tissues. Understanding how and where these enzymes function can provide valuable insight about how dopamine is functioning in specific regions of the body. In order to understand these functions one must first realise that Monoamine oxidase (MAO) is an enzyme present within the cytoplasm of neurons that breaks down dopamine to DOPAL. DOPAL in turn is very rapidly converted to DOPAC by a second cytoplasmic enzyme aldehyde dehydrogenase (AD). Because both of these enzymes are primarily found inside neurons, DOPAC levels are dependent on the amount of cytoplasmic dopamine. Combined measurements of DOPAC and dopamine have been used to assess the activity of dopaminergic neurons. This combination provides additional information than either parameter alone because a large portion of DOPAC is formed from dopamine without ever being released to the synaptic cleft. This suggests that DOPAC may be more closely related to the presynaptic dopamine levels while dopamine and similarly HVA levels, another important metabolite of dopamine that is formed outside of the neuron via the actions of catechols-O-methyltransferase (COMT), are related to the rate of neuron signalling. Said another way, extracellular DOPAC is related to the amount of dopamine made and stored in the presynaptic neuron while extracellular dopamine levels are related to the rate of dopamine released via the depolarisation of dopamine neurons.

DOSAGE
The amount of medicine to be given.

DOUBLE BLIND
A type of scientific experiment in which neither the subjects nor the researchers know who is receiving an active substance and who is receiving a placebo. Researchers who do not know which subjects received the active substance then usually evaluate the data generated from the experiment. This type of experiment helps to eliminate personal bias from research.

ENDOMETRIOSIS
The presence of uterine lining in other pelvic organs, esp. the ovaries, characterised by cyst formation, adhesions and menstrual pains.

ENVIRONMENTAL FACTORS
Those determinants of disease that are not transmitted genetically and may determine the development of disease in those genetically predisposed to a particular condition. Environmental factors include stress, physical and mental abuse, diet, exposure to toxins, pathogens, radiation and chemicals found in almost all personal care products and household cleaners are common environmental factors that determine a large segment of non-hereditary disease.

EPINEPHRINE

Epinephrine, also known as adrenaline, is an excitatory neurotransmitter and hormone essential for lipolysis, which is a process in which the body metabolizes fat. Epinephrine is derived from the amine norepinephrine. As a neurotransmitter, epinephrine regulates attentiveness and mental focus. Epinephrine is synthesized from norepinephrine. As a hormone, epinephrine is secreted along with norepinephrine principally by the medulla of the adrenal gland. Heightened secretion can occur in response to fear or anger and will result in increased heart rate and the hydrolysis of glycogen to glucose.

This reaction, referred to as the 'fight or flight' response, prepares the body for strenuous activity. Epinephrine is used medicinally as a stimulant in cardiac arrest, as a vasoconstrictor in shock, as a bronchodilator and antispasmodic in bronchial asthma, and anaphylaxis. Commonly, epinephrine levels will be low due to adrenal fatigue (a pattern in which the adrenal output is suppressed due to chronic stress). Therefore, symptoms can be presented as fatigue with low epinephrine levels. Low levels of epinephrine can also contribute to weight gain and poor concentration. Elevated levels of epinephrine can be factors contributing to restlessness, anxiety, sleep problems, or acute stress

ERECTILE DYSFUNCTION

Difficulty in achieving or maintaining an erection of the penis; impotence.

ESTRADIOL (SEE OESTRADIOL)

ESTRIOL (SEE OESTRIOL)

ESTRONE (SEE OESTRONE)

FATIGUE

Weariness or exhaustion of the mind or body from labour, exertion, or stress.

FIBROIDS

A benign tumour composed of fibrous or muscle tissue, especially one that develops in the uterus.

FIBROMYALGIA

A syndrome characterised by chronic pain in the muscles and soft tissues surrounding the joints, fatigue and tenderness at specific sites in the body. Also called fibromyalgia syndrome, fibromyositis, fibrositis.

FOLLICLE STIMULATING HORMONE

A gonadotropic hormone of the anterior pituitary gland that stimulates the growth of follicles in the ovary and induces the formation of sperm in the testes.

FORGETFULNESS

Loss of remembrance or recollection; a ceasing to remember. Also called memory loss, foggy thinking, or foggy memory.

FREE RADICALS

Harmful molecules that cause damage in the body; leading factors in the development of blood vessel disease (atherosclerosis), cancer and other conditions. By-products of normal body processes, by-products of the breakdown of certain medicines, found in pollutants.

GABA

GABA is a true neurotransmitter and is the major inhibitory neurotransmitter of the brain, occurring in 30-40% of all synapses. GABA is second only to glutamate, the brain's major excitatory neurotransmitter. The GABA concentration in the brain is 200-1000 times greater than that of the monoamines or acetylcholine. The primary function of GABA is to prevent overstimulation. It does so by compensating for glutamate activity. When GABA activates its receptor it causes negative ions to flow into the cell preventing depolarisation. Glutamate can depolarise the cell and form an action potential by causing positive ions to flow into the cell when it activates its receptors. Overall, GABA regulates the activity of glutamate by preventing depolarization of the cell, therefore, preventing overstimulation.

GALACTORRHEA

Secretion of milk from the breast of a non-lactating person.

GAMMA-AMINOBUTYRIC ACID (GABA)
A neurotransmitter of the central nervous system that inhibits excitatory responses.

GLUTAMATE
Glutamate is the major excitatory neurotransmitter in the brain which is necessary for memory and learning. In fact, it is believed that 70% of the fast excitatory CNS synapses utilize glutamate as a transmitter. Excitatory neurotransmitters increase the activity of signal-receiving neurons and play a major role in controlling brain function. Glutamate exerts its effects on cells, in part, through three types of receptors that, when activated, allow the flow of positively charged ions into the cell. These include the ionotropic receptors: kianate, alpha-amino-3-hydroxy-5-methyl-4-isoxazolepropionic acid (AMPA) and N-methyl-D-aspartate (NMDA) receptors. There are also series metabotropic glutamate receptors that do not directly manipulate an ion channel. Of the ionotropic receptors, the N-methyl-D-aspartate (NMDA) receptor plays a particularly important role in controlling the brain's ability to adapt to environmental and genetic influences which is important for learning and memory.

GLYCINE
Glycine is a principal inhibitory amino acid in the brainstem and spinal cord that regulates excitatory neurotransmission in much the same way as GABA. Glycine, much like GABA and taurine, can become elevated to compensate for elevations in excitatory neurotransmitters, primarily, glutamate and aspartic acid. This non-essential amino acid is common in protein-based foods, and can be synthesised metabolically from a number of different amino acids, including serine and threonine. Curiously, glycine is a necessary cofactor in the activation of the glutamate receptor, NMDA. It seems paradoxical that a primarily inhibitory amino acid facilitates the activation of an excitatory receptor. It has been postulated that glycine's inhibitory and excitatory actions are part of the many checks and balances the body has for regulating neurotransmission.

GROWTH HORMONE (GH)
A hormone secreted by the pituitary gland. GH stimulates growth and repair of the body as well as the activities of the immune system. With age, GH release diminishes (also known as HGH or human growth hormone).

GYNAECOMASTIA
Abnormal enlargement of the breasts in a male.

HAIR LOSS
The medical description of the loss of hair from the head or body, sometimes to the extent of baldness, that is involuntary and unwelcome. In some cases, it is an indication of an underlying medical concern, such as iron deficiency. Also called alopecia.

HEALTH
The general condition of the body or mind with reference to soundness and vigour.

HISTAMINE
An excitatory neurotransmitter involved in the sleep/wake cycle and inflammatory response.

Depending on the receptor, histamine activates a wide array of biological actions can occur. For instance, one receptor helps regulate the sleep/wake cycle whereas another receptor helps regulates norepinephrine, serotonin, and acetylcholine release. There are also other receptors that may be activated to induce inflammatory response, which is commonly associated with the exposure to an allergen.

HORMONE
Latin for a chemical messenger, such as growth hormone, testosterone or insulin.

HORMONE PELLET THERAPY
A sustainable delivery method or treatment option for bio-identical hormone therapy. Every three to six months a pellet made of bio-identical hormones is inserted just under the patient's skin. The pellets, which contain customised levels of oestradiol or testosterone, react to the needs of the body, so they actually dissolve releasing the bio-identical hormones as needed.

HORMONE THERAPY
The use of hormones in medical treatment. Also called hormonal therapy.

HOT FLUSH
A sudden feeling of feverish heat typically as a symptom of menopause. Also called a hot flash.

HYPERTHYROIDISM
Pathologically excessive production of the thyroid hormones.

HYPOGONADISM
Diminished hormonal or reproductive functioning in the testes or the ovaries.

HYPOTHALAMUS
An area of the brain that is believed to be the command centre for instructions to the endocrine system.

HYPOTHYROIDISM
Deficient activity of the thyroid gland.

HYSTERECTOMY
Surgical removal of part or the entire uterus. Also called surgical menopause.

IMBALANCE
Lack of proportion or relation between corresponding things: the condition is caused by a hormone imbalance.

INSOMNIA
Inability to obtain sufficient sleep, especially when chronic; difficulty in falling or staying asleep. Also called sleeplessness.

INTERSTITIAL CYSTITIS
A urinary bladder disease of unknown cause characterised by urinary frequency, urgency, pressure and/or pain in the bladder and/or pelvis. Also known as painful bladder syndrome (PBS).

IODINE
An element required in small amounts for healthy growth and development. The thyroid gland requires iodine to synthesise thyroid hormones; a deficiency of the element leads to goitre.

IRRITABLE
Easily irritated or annoyed; readily excited to impatience or anger.

IRRITABLE MALE SYNDROME
The term for a set of symptoms caused by a drop in testosterone levels in males. These symptoms are similar to those of the male menopause or andropause. One of the most consistent symptoms is anger and sullen withdrawal present in men between the ages of 40 and 60.

LANCET
A small surgical instrument, usually sharp-pointed and two-edged, for making small incisions like opening abscesses.

LIBIDO
Sexual urge or desire.

LONGEVITY
A long individual life; great duration of individual life.

LUTEINIZING HORMONE
A hormone produced by the anterior lobe of the pituitary gland that stimulates ovulation and the development of the corpus luteum in the female and the production of testosterone by the interstitial cells of the testes in the male

LYMPHOCYTES
Any of the various white blood cells, including B-cells and T-cells, that function in the body's immune system by recognising and deactivating specific foreign substances called antigens. B-cells act by stimulating the production of antibodies. T-cells contain receptors on their cell surfaces that are capable of recognizing

and binding to specific antigens. Lymphocytes are found in the lymph nodes and spleen, and circulate continuously in the blood and lymph.

MELATONIN
A hormone derived from serotonin and secreted by the pineal gland in inverse proportion to the amount of light received by the retina. Darkness perceived by the retina (or sleep) induces greater production which has been linked to the regulation of circadian rhythms and inducing sleep rhythms.

MENOPAUSAL
Of, pertaining to, or characteristic of menopause.

MENOPAUSE
The period of permanent cessation of menstruation, usually occurring between the ages of 45 and 55.

MENSTRUAL CYCLE
A recurring cycle in which the endometrial lining of the uterus prepares for pregnancy; if pregnancy does not occur the lining is shed at menstruation. The average menstrual cycle is 28 days, day 1 being the beginning of bleeding.

MENSTRUATION
The periodic discharge of blood and mucosal tissue from the uterus, occurring approximately monthly from puberty to menopause in non-pregnant women.

METABOLIC RATE
The rate of metabolism; the amount of energy expended in a given period.

METABOLISM
The sum of the physical and chemical processes in an organism, by which its material substance is produced, maintained and destroyed and by which energy is made available.

METABOLITES
Substances necessary for taking part in a particular metabolic process, such as glucose in the metabolism of sugars and starches, and amino acids in the biosynthesis of proteins.

MICRONIZED
To reduce to particles only a few microns in diameter.

MIDLIFE CRISIS
A period of psychological stress occurring in middle age, thought to be triggered by a physical, occupational, or domestic event, such as menopause or andropause, diminution of physical prowess, job loss, or departure of children from the home.

MOBILE PHLEBOTOMY
A blood draw or venesection at a different location than the normal doctor's office or laboratory; usually at a patient's home.

MOLECULE
A single very small particle, made up of atoms, which is indivisible.

MOOD SWING(S)
An abrupt and apparently unaccountable change of mood.

NEUROTRANSMITTER
Any of several chemical substances, such as epinephrine or acetylcholine, that transmit nerve impulses across a synapse to a postsynaptic element, such as another nerve, muscle or gland.

NIGHT SWEAT
Copious sweating during sleep. Night sweats may be an early indication of tuberculosis, AIDS, or other disease.

NITRIC OXIDE
Works as a signalling molecule in the cardiovascular system. Cells of a blood vessel's inner walls use nitric oxide to signal the vessel to relax and dilate, increasing blood flow.

NOREPINEPHRINE
Norepinephrine is an excitatory neurotransmitter that is important for attention and focus. Norepinephrine is synthesised from dopamine by means of the enzyme dopamine beta-hydroxylase, with oxygen, copper, and vitamin C as co-factors.

Dopamine is synthesized in the cytoplasm, but norepinephrine is synthesised in the neurotransmitter storage vesicles.

Cells that use norepinephrine for formation of epinephrine use SAMe as a methyl group donor. Levels of epinephrine in the CNS are only about 10% of the levels of norepinephrine.

OBSTRUCTIVE SLEEP APNOEA
Sleep apnoea that is caused by recurring interruption of breathing during sleep because of the obstruction of the upper airway by weak or malformed pharyngeal tissues, that occurs especially in obese middle-aged and elderly men, and that results in hypoxaemia and chronic lethargy during the day. Also called obstructive sleep apnoea syndrome.

OESTRADIOL
The most powerful female hormone that occurs naturally. An oestrogenic hormone produced by the ovaries and used in treating oestrogen deficiency and certain menopausal and postmenopausal conditions.

OESTRIOL
An oestrogenic hormone occurring in urine during pregnancy; used in conditions involving oestrogen deficiency.

OESTROGEN

Any of several steroid hormones produced chiefly by the ovaries and responsible for the development and maintenance of female secondary sex characteristics.

OESTROGEN DOMINANCE

A condition in which a person has excess amounts of oestrogen in the body.

OESTRONE

An oestrogenic hormone produced by the ovarian follicles and found during pregnancy in urine and placental tissue; used in the treatment of oestrogen deficiency and certain menopausal and postmenopausal conditions.

OVER-THE-COUNTER

Sold legally without a doctor's prescription: over-the-counter drugs.

OVULATION

To produce and discharge eggs from an ovary or ovarian follicle.

PARKINSON'S DISEASE

A degenerative disorder of the central nervous system characterized by tremor and impaired muscular coordination.

PEA

Beta-phenylethylamine (PEA) is an excitatory neurotransmitter derived from the amino acid phenylalanine. Studies have found that PEA promotes energy and elevates mood. PEA also functions as a synaptic neuromodulator inhibiting the reuptake of dopamine and norepinephrine. Studies have discovered that patients with depression have decreased PEA levels while increased levels have been found in patients with psychopathic symptoms. It has also been implicated in headaches and the antidepressant effects of exercise. One of the biochemical abnormalities resulting from phenylketonuria, the absence of the enzyme that helps to synthesize phenylalanine into tyrosine, is an increased production of PEA. This can cause an elevated level of PEA in the urine. Since PEA is lipid soluble and readily crosses the blood-brain-barrier, the administration of PEA or of its precursor, phenylalanine, has been found to improve outcome with some antidepressants. Also, supplementation to manipulate PEA can help increase focus and attention.

PERIMENOPAUSE
The period around the onset of menopause that is often marked by various physical changes, such as hot flushes and menstrual irregularity. Also called early menopause or premenopause.

PHLEBOTOMY
The act or practice of opening a vein for letting blood as a therapeutic measure. Also called venesection.

PHYTOESTROGENS
Sometimes called 'dietary estrogens', are a diverse group of naturally occurring non steroidal plant compounds that, because of their structural similarity with oestradiol, have the ability to cause oestrogenic or/and anti-oestrogenic effects.

PITUITARY GLAND
A gland at the base of the brain. The pituitary secretes several different hormones involved in key metabolic processes.

POST MENOPAUSE
All of the time in a woman's life that take place after her last period ever, or more accurately, all of the time that follows the point when her ovaries become inactive. A woman who still has her uterus can be declared to be in post menopause once she has gone 12 full months with no flow at all, not even any spotting. Also seen as postmenopause or post-menopause.

PRECURSOR
A chemical that can be converted by the body into another is a precursor of the latter chemical.

PREGNENOLONE
An unsaturated hydroxyl steroid that is formed by the oxidation of steroids (like cholesterol) and yields progesterone on dehydrogenation.

PREMENSTRUAL SYNDROME (PMS)
A varied group of physical and psychological symptoms, including abdominal bloating, breast tenderness, headache, fatigue, irritability, anxiety and depression that occur from 2 to 7 days before the onset of menstruation and cease shortly after menses begins.

PRESCRIPTION
A direction, usually written by the physician to the pharmacist for the preparation and use of a medicine or remedy.

PREVENTIVE MEDICINE
Measures taken to prevent illness or injury, rather than curing them. Preventive care may include examinations and screening tests tailored to an individual's age, health and family history. Also called preventive care or preventative medicine.

PROGESTERONE
A hormone that prepares the uterus for the fertilised ovum and maintains pregnancy.

PROLACTIN
A protein hormone produced by the pituitary gland of mammals that acts with other hormones to initiate the secretion of milk by the mammary glands. It also acts to maintain the corpus luteum of the ovary, which is the source of the female sex hormone progesterone. In males, high levels of prolactin can cause testosterone levels to decrease.

PROSTATE SPECIFIC ANTIGEN (PSA)
A protein produced by the cells of the prostate gland. PSA is present in small quantities in the serum of normal men and is often elevated in the presence of prostate cancer and in other prostate disorders.

RECEPTORS

A molecular structure or site on the surface or interior of a cell that binds with substances such as hormones.

REVERSE TRIIODOTHYRONINE (REVERSE T3)

A molecule which is an isomer of triiodothyroniine and derived from thyroxine through the use of deiodinase. Blocks the action of T3.

SELF-INJECTION

The act of injecting oneself with a drug or other substance.

SEROTONIN

Serotonin is an inhibitory neurotransmitter synthesised by enzymes that act on tryptophan and/or 5-HTP. Serotonin is stored in presynaptic vesicles and released to transmit electrochemical signals across the synapse. Extensive research has been conducted surrounding serotonin which acts as a target for symptoms like low mood, compulsions, anxiousness, and headaches. Serotonin acts, in most cases, as an inhibitory neurotransmitter and, like GABA, modulates neuron voltage potentials to inhibit glutamate activity and neurotransmitter firing. Serotonin neurons have large numbers of axons and are important in integrating neural circuits. This also provides an explanation for serotonin's role in so many health concerns. An inhibitory neurotransmitter required for sleep.

SEROTONIN METABOLITE

5-Hydroxyindoleacetic acid (5-HIAA) is a major metabolite of serotonin, generated via a two-step process, involving monoamine oxidase A (MAO-A) and aldehyde dehydrogenase. Measurement of 5-HIAA in combination with serotonin may offer insight into mechanisms underlying various clinical symptoms. The ratio of serotonin to 5-HIAA may be used to evaluate serotonin turnover and monoamine oxidase activity. Abnormal levels of 5-HIAA have been associated with depression, suicidal behaviours, aggression, chronic psychotropic medication use, and Parkinson's Disease.

SERUM

The clear yellowish fluid obtained upon separating whole blood into its solid and liquid components after it has been allowed to clot.

SEX DRIVE

A physiological need for sexual activity.

SEX HORMONE

Any of a class of steroid hormones that regulate the growth and function of the reproductive organs or stimulate the development of the secondary sexual characteristics.

SEX HORMONE-BINDING GLOBULIN (SHBG)

A glycoprotein produced by the liver cells that binds to sex hormones, specifically testosterone and oestradiol.

SLEEP APNOEA

A temporary suspension of breathing occurring repeatedly during sleep that is caused especially by obstruction of the airway or a disturbance in the brain's respiratory centre and is associated especially with excessive daytime sleepiness.

STEROID HORMONES

Any hormone containing the characteristic steroid ring complex; a term often associated with hormones such as progesterone, testosterone, oestrogens, DHEA, and others.

STRESS

Physical, mental, or emotional strain or tension; a specific response by the body to stimulus, as fear or pain, that disturbs or interferes with the normal physiological equilibrium of an organism.

STRESSORS

An agent, condition or other stimulus that causes stress to an organism.

SYMPTOM(S)

A subjective indication of a disorder reported by an afflicted person rather than being observed by an examiner.

SYNTHETIC HORMONES

Hormones made from plant progesterone and animal chemicals that are bio-similar but not identical to the hormones your body uses. Generally, an extra covalent bond or molecules are added so that it can be patented or to alter its chemical properties or clinical effects. Being non-identical to the body may cause significant harmful side effects.

TAURINE

Taurine is an inhibitory neurotransmitter involved in neuro modulatory and neuroprotective actions. Supplementing with taurine can have a specific effect on GABA function. There are two primary ways in which taurine affects GABA: First, it can inhibit GABA transaminase, an enzyme that metabolises GABA. This allows GABA to stay in the synaptic cleft longer to bind to the postsynaptic receptor. Second, taurine can bind to the GABAA receptor mimicking the effects of GABA.

By helping GABA function, taurine is an important neuromodulator for prevention of excitoxicity. Excitability occurs when glutamate binds to its receptor, in this case, the NMDA receptor. Once glutamate activates the NMDA receptor there is an increase in intracellular Ca^{++} causing depolarisation or cell excitability. With glutamate release, there is also simultaneous GABA and taurine release. When the inhibitory neurotransmitters, GABA and taurine, activate the GABAA receptor, the result is an increase in intracellular Cl- ions. This results in hyperpolarisation which reduces cell excitability. Thus, the overall effect of taurine supplementation is to support GABA function. The relevance of GABA support is to prevent over-stimulation due to high levels of excitatory amino acids. Therefore, taurine and GABA constitute an important protective mechanism against excessive excitatory amino acids. Similarly, taurine is increased in response to the exposure of free radicals elucidating its neuroprotective actions. Exposure to free radicals increases glutamate excretion, further potentiation NMDA receptor activation. Taurine modulates this effect to prevent cell excitability by keeping the cell hyperpolarised.

The supplementation of taurine can help alleviate some excitability issues associated with elevated excitatory amino acids as well as play a role in regulating the effect of free radicals.

TESTOSTERONE
A potent Androgenic hormone produced chiefly by the testes, which stimulates the development of male sex organs, secondary sexual traits and sperm.

THYROID
The gland located in the centre and anterior aspect of the neck responsible (amongst other things) for temperature regulation.

THYROID PEROXIDASE (TPO)
An enzyme mainly expressed in the thyroid that liberates iodine for addition onto tyrosine residues on thyroglobulin for the production of T4, T3 and reverse T3.

THYROID STIMULATING HORMONE (TSH)
A glycoprotein hormone secreted by the anterior portion of the pituitary gland that stimulates and regulates the activity of the thyroid gland. Also called thyrotropin.

THYROXIN (T4)
The thyroid gland iodine-containing hormone that regulates the metabolic rate of the body; used in the treatment of hypothyroidism.

TRANSFERRIN
A blood plasma protein for iron ion delivery.

TRIODOTHYRONINE (T3)
A thyroid hormone derived from thyroxine but several times more potent; used in treating hypothyroidism.

TYRAMINE

Tyramine (4-hydroxy-phenethylamine) is a naturally occurring monoamine compound formed by the enzymatic decarboxylation of the aromatic amino acid tyrosine. The enzyme monoamine oxidase is responsible for the breakdown of tyramine. When this metabolic pathway is compromised by monoamine oxidase inhibitors (MAOIs), tyramine levels can become elevated and cause the release of neurotransmitters, such as dopamine, norepinephrine, and epinephrine, potentially leading to an increase in blood pressure. Dietary intake of tyramine has also been associated with cluster headaches and migraines, forcing many to restrict foods containing tyramine such as fish, chocolate, alcohol, and fermented foods including cheese, processed meat, and sauerkraut.

URINARY INCONTINENCE

Any involuntary leakage of urine.

VAGINAL ATROPHY

Loss of muscle tension in the vagina.

VAGINAL DRYNESS

The condition in which vaginal lubrication is insufficient causing increased friction and discomfort during sexual intercourse.

VAGINAL LUBRICATION

The naturally produced lubricating fluid that reduces friction during sexual intercourse.

XENOESTROGEN

Substances or pollutants originating outside the body that have oestrogen-like activities. Exposure to these substances can have a profound impact on a person's natural hormonal balance.

XENOHORMONES

Substances or pollutants originating outside the body that have hormone-like activities. Exposure to these substances can have a profound impact on a person's natural hormonal balance.

References

GLUCK, M., V. EDGSON .2010. It must be my hormones. Australia: Penguin Group

LEMMON H. M.; Pathophysiologic consideration in the treatment of menopausal patients with oestrogens; the role of estriol in the prevention of mammary carcinoma; Acta Endocrinol (copenh) 1980; 223:S17-S27)

LABRIE, F., A. DUPONT & A. BELANGER. 1985. Complete androgen blockade for the treatment of prostate cancer. In Important Advances in Oncology, V.T. de Vita, S. Hellman & S.A. Rosenburg, Eds-193-217. J.B. Lippincott, Philadelphia.

BELANGER, A., M. BROCHU & J. CLICH, 1986. Levels of plasma steroid glucuronides in intact and castrated men with prostate cancer. J. Clin. Endocrinal Metab. 62:812-815.

LABRIE, F., A. BELANGER, A. DUPONT, V. LULU-THE, J. SIMARD & C. LABRIE. 1993. Science behind total androgen blockade: From gene to combination therapy. Clin. Invest. Med. 16:487-504.

MOGHISSI, E., F. ABLAN & R. HORTON. 1984. Origin of plasma and androstanediol glucuronide in men. J. Clin. Endocrinol. Metab. 39:417-421

LABRIE, F. 1991. Intracrinology. Mel. Cell. Endrocrinol. 78:C113-C118.

BIRD, C.E., J. MURPHY, K. BOOROOMAND, W. FINNIS, D. DRESSEL & A.F. CLARK. 1978. Dehydroepiandrosterone: Kinetics of metabolism in normal men and women. J. Clin. Endocrinol. Metab. 47:818-822

PLAGER, J.E. 1965. The binding of androsterone sulfate, etiocholanolons sulfate and dehydroisoandrosterone sulfate by human plasma protein. J. Clin. Invest. 44:1234-1239

WANG, D.Y. 7 R.D. BULBROOK. 1967. Binding of the sulphate esters of dehydrepiandrosterone, testosterone, 17-acetoxypregnendlone and pregnenolone in the plasma of man, rabbit, and rat. J. Clin. Endocrinol. 39:405-413

DE NEVE, L. & A. VERMEULEN. 1965. The determination of 17 oxosteroidsulfates in human plasma. J. Endocrinol. 32:295-302

ORENTREICH, N., J.L. BRIND, R. L. RIZER & J.H. VOGELMAN. 1984. Age changes and sex differences in serum dehydroepiandrosterone sulfate concentration during adulthood. J. Clin. Endocrinol. Metab. 59:551-555.

BELANGER, A., B. CARRIDAS, A. DUPONT, L. CUSAN, P. DIAMOND, J.L. GOMEZ 8 F. LABRIE. 1994. Changes in serum concentration of conjugated and unconjugated steroids in 40 to 80 year old men. J. Clin. Endocrinol. Metab.79:1086-1090.

FIELD, A.E., G.EI COLDITZ, W.C. WILLETT, C. LONCOPE & J.B. MCKINLAY. 1994. The relation of smoking, age, relative weight and dietary intake to serum adrenal steroids, sex hormones and sex hormone binding globulin in middle age men. J. Clin. Endocrinol. Metab. 79:1310-1316.

VERMEUULEN, A. 1980. Adrenal androgens and aging. In Adrenal Adrogens, A.R. Genazzani, J.H.H. Thyssen & P.R. Siiteri, Eds. 201-217. Academic Press.

HORNSBY, PETER J., ·1995. Current Challenges for DHEA Research. Annals of the New York Academy of Sciences, Vol.774:xii-xiv.

MORALES, A.J., J.J. NJOLAN, J.C. NELSON & S.S.C. YEN. 1994. Effects of replacement dose of dehydroepiandrosterone in men and women of advancing age. J. Clin. Endocrinol. Metab. 78:1360-1367.

YEN, S.S.C., MORALES, A.J. & KHORRAM, O. 1995. Replacement of DHEA in Aging Men and Women. Annals of the New York Academy of Sciences. Vol.774:128-142.

ORENTREICH, N., J.L. BRIND, R. L. RIZER & J.H. VOGELMAN. 1984. Age changes and sex differences in serum dehydroepiandrosterone sulfate concentration during adulthood. J. Clin. Endocrjnol. Metab. 59:551-555.

CARLSTROM, K., S. BRODY, N.O. LUNELL, A. LAGRELIUS, G. MOLLERSTROM, A. POUSETTE, G. RANNEVIK, R. STEGE & B. VON SCHOULTZ. 1988. Dehydroepiandrosterone in serum: Differences related to age and sex. Maturitas 10:297-306.

ORENTREICH, N., J.L. BRIND, J.H. VOGELMAN, RR. ANDRES & H. BALDWIN. 1992. Long-term longitudinal measurements of plasma Dehydroepiandrosterone sulfate in normal men. J. Clin. Endocrinol. Metab. 75:1002-1004.

Reference: Lemmon, HM; Pathophysiologic consideration in the treatment of menopausal patients with oestrogens; the role of estriol in the prevention of mammary carcinoma; Acta Endocrinol (copenh) 1980; 223:S17-S27)